For Hearing People

ONLY

For Hearing People

ONLY

Answers to Some of the
Most Commonly Asked Questions
About the Deaf Community,
its Culture, and the "Deaf Reality"

Second Edition
a newly-revised and expanded compilation
from the popular monthly magazine
DEAF LIFE

by
Matthew S. Moore
and Linda Levitan
Co-Editors-in-Chief
DEAF LIFE

With a foreword by Harlan Lane,
author of **When the Mind Hears: A History of the Deaf** and
The Mask of Benevolence: Disabling the Deaf Community

Deaf Life Press
a division of MSM Productions, Ltd.
Rochester, New York
1993

Cover Design: Dyam Design
Illustrations: Robert L. Johnson
Manual-alphabet capitals: Tony Landon McGregor

Grateful acknowledgement is made to the following: Gallaudet University Press for permission to quote or cite passages from **American Sign Language: A Student Text** by Dennis Cokely and Charlotte Baker; **Ben's Story: A Deaf Child's Right to Sign** by Lorraine Fletcher; **The Other Side of Silence** by Arden Neisser; **I Didn't Hear the Dragon Roar** by Frances M. Parsons; and **A Place of Their Own** by John V. Van Cleve and Barry Crouch; to McGraw-Hill Company for permission to quote a passage from the **Gallaudet Encyclopedia of Deaf People and Deafness**; and to the following individuals whose letters, articles, or comments originally appeared in **DEAF LIFE**: David Anthony; Barb and John Boelter; Paulette Caswell; Duane King; Dr. Richard Nowell; Dr. Peter Seiler; Dr. Allen Sussman; and Dr. Sherman Wilcox. Quotations from **When the Mind Hears** by Harlan Lane are used by permission of the author.

Publisher's Cataloging in Publication Data
Moore, Matthew S., 1958-
Levitan, Linda J., 1951-

For hearing people only: answers to some of the most commonly asked questions about the Deaf community, its culture, and the "Deaf Reality" / Matthew S. Moore and Linda Levitan. With a foreword by Harlan Lane.

Bibliography: p.
Includes index.
ISBN 0-9634016-1-0 (paperback)
1. Deaf studies. 2. Deaf—Culture. 3. Deaf—United States—background. 4. Sign language. I. Title.

                                                                            93-90673
                                                                                 CIP

Printed in the United States of America

The paper use in this publication meets the minimum requirements of American National Standard for Information Sciences—Permanence of Paper for Printed Library Materials, ANSI Z39.48-1984 (∞)

10 9 8 7 6 5 4 3 2
Second Edition

1st Printing, 8/1993	6th Printing, 2/1997	11th Printing, 2/2001
2nd Printing, 1/1994	7th Printing, 12/1997	12th Printing, 12/2001
3rd Printing, 6/1994	8th Printing, 11/1998	
4th Printing, 7/1995	9th Printing, 9/1999	
5th Printing, 5/1996	10th Printing, 7/2000	

For all hearing people who want to better
understand our community and our language,
and for all those, deaf and hearing,
who helped make this book possible.

For my mother, JoNelle, who sought out
the best education for me;
for Tom Connor, Jr., my best friend,
for allowing me to be me;
and for Charles Francis Bancroft—
T.R.A.G. and D.F.S.S. now and forever!
—MSM

For my parents, in the hope that
they will *finally* understand;
for my good teachers, counselors, and friends—
particularly Dante Ippolito, Olga Veckys, Gary Roy,
Dawn Goodrich, Karen Johnsen,
Tina Salvo, Liz Shaw, and Mac Sintes;
for all those who have shown me that
"living well is the *best* revenge;"
and, especially, for my boss, who taught me
something about "thinking positive."
—LL

And to the memory of all those deaf people
who died because of failed or inaccessible
communications, misunderstandings,
and ignorance on the part of society.

Foreword

I doubt whether people are more curious about anything in life than other people—especially other people with another culture. Imagine for a moment striking all discussion of how other groups act, think, socialize, and view the world from conversation, literature and the other arts (not to mention travel books); really, what would we talk about? How many of our sentences start something like: "Although the Germans . . ." "The thing about people from California . . ." "Despite the way Japanese people . . ." For many years, I resisted. French people, I said, are so different one to the next that I refuse to generalize. (Besides, the stereotypes were either adoring or totally damning and neither extreme was plausible.) But in the end I had to give in and generalize—I found I was being left out of too many conversations.

The trouble is, these descriptions of people with another culture are rarely unbiased and rarely well-informed. You are told that French people are unfriendly, Japanese self-effacing, Deaf clannish; what you are not told is: I feel more comfortable in familiar surroundings; I didn't know how to read the taxi meter; I had no idea how to begin politely; I couldn't communicate well enough to be interesting. (If only people said what they meant and meant what they said!) The problem, in my opinion, is that we have too much hasty and deceptive description of others and not enough self-description.

This is especially true for relatively invisible cultures like Deaf culture. How are outsiders to learn about it—to learn even the rudiments; for example, that there *is* such a culture? I think the members of the Deaf community may fail to appreciate how utterly unaware hearing people are of the existence of their culture. (The published remarks of some distinguished Deaf people denying that there is such a culture have not helped.) There is, after all, no Chinatown or Little Italy of the Deaf. Until recently, the language of the Deaf community was not taught in our high schools and colleges. (That has changed dramatically but the language is still grudgingly granted second-class status in most schools.) Deaf culture is rarely portrayed in the media, as infrequently as Black, Native American or Gay culture was portrayed when I was a boy.

There is a special obstacle to hearing people's understanding of Deaf culture in particular. Whereas few Americans construct for themselves an image of Hispanic culture (for example) by extrapolating—by imagining themselves with mastery of their high-school Spanish and a meal ticket to Taco Bell—most Americans who are led to think about Deaf culture do construct their idea of the lives of Deaf people by extrapolating—by imagining themselves without hearing. Of course, a real difference in culture does not enter into this equation (only abrupt silence, a loss, not a gain) and so it is utterly useless to solve any problem that concerns culturally Deaf people. This acultural approach to Deaf culture leaves hearing people with only the concept of handicap to guide them.

Although we never tire of figuring out what the other person can't do, we are almost invariably wrong. Blacks, women and gays couldn't fight alongside straight white males; a deaf person could not be a major actress, lawyer, doctor. We underestimate human ingenuity— and thus ourselves. The same flexibility (miraculous plasticity, really) that fosters spoken languages in hearing people and signed languages in visual people, fosters novel solutions to many of life's challenges. Then, too, "can't" can be a self-fulfilling prophecy. The only clear human "can't" is—you can't figure out most of the time what someone very different from yourself can and cannot do.

Alas, uninformed guesses at what deafness must be like are frequently presented as authoritative by hearing people who stand to gain by such pronouncements. There is a vast literature on "the Deaf"—countless journals, books, texts, theses, etc. (I review it critically in my new book, **The Mask of Benevolence: Disabling the Deaf Community**.) This is the record mostly of hearing people explaining their ideas about deafness to other hearing people. It has many false stereotypes; it suffers from ignorance of ASL and Deaf culture and Deaf history; it is as bad for what it fails to say (about Deaf art, for example) as for what it does say (about Deaf thought). It is about as useful as Europeans' explanations to each other about what Africans are really like. It is, however, more dangerous because it is presented as the product of social science research.

Hearing people's account of Deaf people is, then, very faulty, yet our government listens exclusively to hearing people in matters concerning Deaf people. Only hearing people at the Food and Drug Administration decided to approve cochlear implants for young deaf children (down to the age of two). Only hearing people at the National Institute on Deafness and Other Communication Disorders [sic] decide on what research should be conducted concerning the Deaf community, ASL, Deaf literacy, Deaf heredity, and much more. Only hearing people in the Department of Education refuse to provide ASL-using children with the special bilingual programs provided children from other language minorities.

So we need more self-description by Deaf people

(among other cultural groups) and I think outsiders would ask for such descriptions more often if we were not so afraid of appearing the fool or of offending. There are two kinds of questions we are tempted to ask, if we only dared. The first kind satisfies our curiosity about obvious differences. I recall an African friend arriving in Boston at midnight on his first trip abroad. As we left the airport, we encountered a few other cars on the highway. "Where is everybody going?" he asked. A question of this first type addressed to Deaf people might be: Is there one universal sign language for Deaf people?

The second kind of question, harder to formulate (why haven't anthropologists helped us more here?), concerns carving an unfamiliar fowl at the joints. What are the revealing questions to ask? We want to know whether the other group, so startlingly different on the surface, doesn't really see the world much as we do and, if not, how its vision differs. Is there another (better?) way to conceive and manage intimacy? Decision making? Spirituality? Wealth? What constitutes achievement? Great art? A good life? These are the more interesting issues, but if we ask any questions at all we are more likely to ask the first kind, the easy ones. And perhaps, after all, those elementary matters need to be cleared up first.

Deaf people have long been trying to explain themselves to hearing people if we would only listen. The first published trace may be Pierre Desloges' well-known book, published in Paris in 1779, where he defends French Sign Language against the false claims of its detractors, hearing teachers who didn't know the least bit about it. The first traces of this self-description in America may be Laurent Clerc's public speeches throughout the northeastern United States, reprinted in the newspapers in 1816. Ever since, there has been a great tradition of Deaf self-description through art, drama, poetry, literature and nonfiction. Just a few examples of the latter are **The Silent Worker**, **A Deaf Adult Speaks Out**, **Deaf Heritage**, **DEAF LIFE** and now this book, **For Hearing People Only**.

In one sense the Deaf culture reflected in **For Hearing People Only** is unfamiliar—in another it is thoroughly familiar. Take language, for example. Sign Language is in an unfamiliar mode (visual and manual, not aural and oral) and it works in unexpected ways. But hearing people will find the puns, jokes, slang, highfalutin language, putdowns, tall tales and so on, familiar to them from their own language. Or, consider the Deaf club. In the neighborhood of Brooklyn where I grew up there were many ethnic clubs. For example, there was a Polish-American club over a nearby supermarket, its name stenciled in black on the windows. Many evenings when the subway brought me home from high school I looked across from the elevated station into the club and saw men in rolled-up shirtsleeves playing cards, thick plumes of purple smoke rising from their cigars. Sometimes I would pass them on the street as a handful would enter or leave the building. They had their own mysterious language, their own camaraderie—that much was clear. They had dances and parties, too (at those times, women were invited). I am reminded of all this on Las Vegas Night at the Boston Deaf Club.

For Hearing People Only contains the responses of the editors of **DEAF LIFE** to questions submitted by their hearing readers. Sincere questions deserve straight answers and that's what the reader will find here. Good common sense. Opinion backed by scholarship. Pride in Deaf culture. A sense of humor. The topics range over language (How do Deaf people learn ASL?), parenting (Is it better to be a hearing child of Deaf parents or a Deaf child of hearing parents?), history (Was Alexander Graham Bell as much of a villain as he appears to have been?), relations with hearing people (Why don't Deaf people trust them?)—and much, much more. How do hearing people come off in this Deaf cultural document? I have told how hearing people commonly describe Deaf people in unflattering terms—well, the compliment is returned! We are seen as woefully ignorant—prey to the most ridiculous beliefs: Deaf people can't drive well, shouldn't marry one another, they speak a universal language, read Braille, can't dance . . . In the last chapter Deaf readers sound off with gripes of their own about hearing people. They accuse us hearing people of having a low opinion of them and revealing it in our actions and our words. We rudely leave them out of conversation. We change our manner of speaking and exaggerate it when we learn someone is deaf, making lipreading more difficult. We expect Deaf people to perform on our terms and never we on theirs.

There is much for hearing people to learn here and much for us to reflect on. **For Hearing People Only** will interest anyone with a connection to Deaf people, of course—parents, teachers, co-workers, students of ASL, to name a few—but, more broadly, it will entertain and inform everyone who rejoices at the rich diversity of humankind and sees in its examination an opportunity to glimpse our essential humanity and to live a more considered life.

Harlan Lane

Acknowledgements

First of all, our profound thanks to those readers of **DEAF LIFE**, whether Deaf, deaf, hard-of-hearing, or hearing, who sent us their thoughtful and provocative questions—sometimes in multiples. (They have provided some of the answers as well.) We are grateful to the National Information Center on Deafness at Gallaudet University for supplying resource information, contacts, articles, and answers to some of the questions.

Harlan Lane, Dr. Robert Panara, Dr. Frank Turk, and Leslie C. Greer generously gave their time to read through the manuscript. Dr. Lane took time from an extraordinarily busy schedule to provide a foreword. We valued their comments, criticisms, and suggestions.

Charles F. Bancroft (the other member of the **DEAF LIFE** team) provided input, assisted with the essential legwork, and helped see us through the inevitable computer foul-ups and catastrophes.

Any errors are our own.

Table of Contents

Introduction

This book is inspired by and written for hearing people who have questions about Deaf culture, sign language, and Deaf life in general, and need a quick answer. It is not intended to be an in-depth excursion into a vast and complex subject, but it may provide accurate and provocative answers to at least some persistent questions. Our scope is necessarily limited; we want our answers to be as concise and accessible as possible to every reader, no matter how limited their background.

Each chapter is designed as an independent unit focusing on one topic. Although we have tried to keep repetition to a minimum, there is an inevitable amount of overlap. Certain facts, we found, needed to be restated.

We have written the monthly installments of "For Hearing People Only" in **DEAF LIFE**, and have compiled this book, with our families and friends in mind—as well as beginning students of ASL and the casual reader who's taking a peek into this subject for the first time. It can be used as a handy in-class or supplementary text in beginning ASL or Deaf Studies classes.

For Hearing People Only is written by two Deaf persons. One is congenitally deaf, a native ASL signer, educated at a school for the deaf, and bilingual. The other is progressively deafened and has personally experienced being hearing, hard-of-hearing, moderately, *and* (currently) severely-deaf-on-the-left, profoundly-deaf-on-the-right—the whole shebang. The illustrators, Tony Landon McGregor and Robert L. Johnson, are both Deaf.

About the terminology used in this book: We wish to de-emphasize the concept of "deafness" and emphasize "the Deaf reality." Even such a seemingly neutral term as "deafness" can have a faintly negative connotation. There are two basic ways of looking at deafness: medically and culturally. The medical view sees deaf people in terms of deficit—broken, wounded, malfunctioning, or disordered ears. The cultural view sees deaf people as persons. Medically speaking, a deaf person has a disability and needs auxiliary aids or surgical intervention to become more "normal." Culturally speaking, to be deaf is to be whole, and thus, different but every bit as "normal." We have a language; we have an identity; we have gifts. We often capitalize the "D" in "deaf" to emphasize this cultural affiliation and pride as members of a sign-language-using community. We use the word "deaf" with a small "d" in the broader sense— medically deaf, but not necessarily culturally-Deaf. Likewise, we will occasionally capitalize the "H" in "hearing" to emphasize the cultural aspect of the surrounding society, the hearing majority.

Why did we title this book **For Hearing People Only**? Hearing people—those with normal hearing—do not think of themselves as being "hearing people." They think of themselves as, well, people. You are the insiders. To you, we deaf people are the outsiders. You call us "deaf people." But we deaf people see non-deaf people as the outsiders—"hearing people." We are a minority with an ancient history of oppression. And oppression is signified by labels. It was Aristotle who first started labeling us "deaf and dumb." Thousands of years later, we are still struggling to free ourselves from that label. To deaf people, the non-deaf majority are "hearing people." The labeled minority has its own label for the labeling majority. As a label, "hearing" can have negative or positive connotations, just as "deaf" does in common (Hearing) usage.

We hope it makes our readers think twice about images—the image you have of deaf people, and the images deaf people have of you. It will, we hope, shake some readers' minds up a bit.

It can be said with reasonable certainty that Deaf people have a far better understanding of the majority ("Hearing") culture that surrounds them than hearing people have of Deaf culture. Deaf people can hardly fail to grasp it; they're bombarded with it from all sides from the time they're born. Not so with hearing people. The Deaf world has long been a closed community, an invisible walled city—an alien and mysterious place many people refused to concede existed at all. Most "Hearing" images of it have been highly distorted. Even today, we find an earthly abundance of misunderstandings, stereotypes, skewed perceptions, and just plain ignorance about deaf people. Books, newspapers, magazines, movies, plays, TV programs—all are powerful tools for shaping opinions, but all have served to perpetuate erroneous ideas about our culture, language, and our abilities as individuals.

We began monthly publication of **DEAF LIFE** in July 1988. From the beginning, we recognized the need to include an informative column written especially for our hearing readers—to mix our metaphors—a palatable morsel of information offered in a way that respects their intelligence while steering them away from prejudicial ways of thinking. It has become one of our most enduringly popular features—perhaps *the* most popular.

"Do you read lips?" "Don't all deaf people read lips?" "Do all deaf people use the same sign language?" "If you're deaf, how come you can talk?" "Can deaf people hear at all?" "Is sign language like Braille?" "Who invented sign language?" These are questions we've run into again and again. We've gotten them from children, teenagers, and adults of all manner of backgrounds—even our own parents. The prevalence of such questions emphasizes the need to educate everyone in at least a basic grasp of Deaf culture. All the questions in this book have been sent to us, asked directly of us, or are based on questions we've encountered (in books, for example). Individual readers have sent in a number of these questions—about communication, attitudes, Deaf history, medical aspects of deafness, education, and linguistic aspects of sign language. We've gotten some exceptionally good and difficult questions from a teacher at Bakersfield College in California who solicited questions from her 150 sign-language students and sent us the 10 best. Some questions, of course, are far more difficult to answer than others. We cherish them all and seek to give them the best answers we can. (Some we have turned over to our readers, especially deaf ones. Our title notwithstanding, we know that deaf people read "HPO," and this book is for them, too.)

Smart people can ask dumb questions, but "dumb" questions aren't necessarily dumb—and all questions deserve good answers. Those who ask questions are at least *thinking* about the subject, even momentarily; at least they're *asking*. The truly apathetic ones have no questions at all. They are our real problems. We hope that at least some of them may find their way to this book. With each step forward, each spurt of shared understanding and enlightenment, each tiny victory, we are constantly reminded that we still have a long distance to cover. **For Hearing People Only** is intended as a small contribution towards that effort.

We wish our readers a good browse. If you are left with more questions than answers, feel free to share them with us! We plan to publish periodic updated sequels to this book. As long as people ask questions about the Deaf community, we will try to meet that need.

Matthew S. Moore
Linda Levitan
Co-Editors-in-Chief, **DEAF LIFE**

Rochester, New York
August 1992

Introduction to the Second Edition

The first edition of this book sold out before June 1993. (Ample proof, we suppose, that it's popular and fills a definite need.) It is with great pleasure that we present the second edition. It contains 12 new chapters adapted from the regular "HPO" installments in the July 1992 through June 1993 issues of **DEAF LIFE**. We've also included the complete "Twelve Faces" cover story ("What do others call us? And what do we call ourselves?") from our May 1993 issue as an addendum to Chapter 25, which deals with labels, terminology, and underlying attitudes.

We wish to thank the many people—individual readers, wholesalers, bookstore staffers, librarians, sign-language teachers, and students—who (to use a mercantile metaphor) were responsible for the rapid turnover of the merchandise, and have kept us hopping for the past year. Thanks for your support! Never a dull moment.

July 1993

Chapter 1

What is ASL?

merican Sign Language (also called ASL or, inaccurately, "Ameslan") is not "bad English," "broken English," "short English," or *any* kind of English. Nor is it Morse Code, or fingerspelling, or pantomime. ASL is a unique language with its own grammatical rules and syntax (sentence structure), and is every bit as precise, versatile, and subtle as English. In some ways, it's even more so.

It's easy enough to describe what ASL isn't. But there is no satisfactory definition of exactly what ASL *is*. Some Deaf people maintain that there can be no universally acceptable, satisfactory-to-all definition of ASL; others claim that there is (or can be). This is a subject of some controversy. Where to draw the line between what's acceptable and unacceptable ASL? Every user seems to have a different opinion!

ASL has evolved from a blend of Old French Sign Language and what's now called "Old American Sign Language," which has been traced to the "dialect" used in the communities of Chilmark and West Tisbury on Martha's Vineyard. Some sort of native sign language was being used well over a century before Laurent Clerc brought French Sign Language to the States in 1817.* ASL, in other words, is a hybrid of FSL and an indigenous sign language. Many ASL signs were borrowed from FSL, but some have always been "American."

At any rate, ASL has developed quite independently of English. Its structure and vocabulary owe nothing to English, or to British Sign Language. Just like any other modern, living and ever-changing language, ASL continues to evolve. Iconic (pictorial or mime-like) signs gradually become more abstract, more arbitrary. New signs are gradually introduced; old signs are altered or dropped. ASL possesses regional variations (dialects), slang, and fad expressions. There are also puns, word-play (like handshape-rhymes), and plenty of creative humor.

ASL has been the precious heritage of the Deaf community, whose users have nonetheless suffered from widespread prejudice in the Hearing world. Not so long ago, Deaf children were discouraged (if not *prohibited*) from using ASL even in schools for the deaf, and adults were ashamed to be seen Signing in public. They were made to feel that ASL was strictly inferior to English, and communicating in Sign was not socially acceptable. (Some "well-meaning" hearing teachers considered it "animal-like."). Happily, we've made progress against such destructively ignorant attitudes, but sentiment against ASL still exists, and deaf children still are discouraged from making ASL their first language.

Linguists have only recently begun to pay serious attention to ASL as a language, but ASL has already begun to enrich American culture through theatre, poetry, song, Sign Mime, and storytelling. A new ASL literature-on-videotape is in the making. Even to those who don't understand it, ASL can be enthralling to watch. Its popularity is steadily increasing, and it has been (arguably) labeled the third most widely-used language in the United States. ASL is a beautiful and expressive language that is finally beginning to get the respect it deserves.

Did you know that...

—people using ASL can communicate comfortably with each other across a football field—much farther than the loudest shout can carry!?

—Sign Language is so handy it's used in underwater communication?

—while whispering can be picked up by microscopic "bugging" devices, sign language is bug-proof? (CIA, take notice!)

—gorillas (and chimpanzees, to some extent) have been taught how to communicate in Sign? (Paradoxically, those who support its use by animals may not favor its use by humans!)

*These communities in Martha's Vineyard had an unusually high incidence of hereditary deafness for many generations. Not only did deaf and hearing residents use Sign with each other, but hearing residents used it among themselves when no deaf people were around. Clerc (1785-1869) was the first Deaf teacher of the deaf in the United States, and co-founder of the American School for the Deaf at Hartford, Connecticut, the first school of its kind here.

How ASL and Deaf Education Began Here (a reasonably brief history)

Deaf people in the American colonies and the early United States, as we've already noted, were using sign language long before 1817.

The history of ASL in the classroom begins in Hartford, Connecticut, in the early 19th century. Dr. Mason Fitch Cogswell, alumnus of Yale, a wealthy and respected physician, had a daughter, Alice (born 1805), who had been early deafened by spotted fever (cerebrospinal meningitis). She was his favorite child. In those days, if you lived in the States and could afford it, you had two options: you sent your child overseas to the famous Braidwood Academy in Edinburgh, Scotland (later London and Manchester, England), or hired a private tutor to teach your child to speak, read, and write. If you were poor, you could keep your child at home or send her/him to an asylum. (No education involved.)

Cogswell could certainly have afforded to send Alice to the Braidwood school, but he undoubtedly recoiled from the idea of shipping her off on the hazardous month-long voyage across the Atlantic Ocean to a foreign country for several years on end. Who could guarantee that he would ever see her again? But he could not find a qualified tutor for her. As for the other alternative—to have her institutionalized ("put away")—he refused to consider it. Alice was obviously bright, but her intellect was not developing normally. She had no real language. There had to be a better way.

Cogswell equipped himself with whatever books he could find on education of the deaf, including one written by the Abbé Sicard, who headed the French Institution Nationale des Sourds-Muets (National Institution for Deaf-Mutes) in Paris. So he knew something about the possibility of education in Sign.

Providentially, Cogswell's neighbors were the Gallaudets, a distinguished merchant family. Thomas Hopkins Gallaudet (b. 1787), also a graduate of Yale and a divinity student, was home recuperating from his chronic ill-health. He happened to notice 9-year-old Alice Cogswell, still languageless, standing apart from the other children, unable to share in their play. For all his fundamentalist fire-and-brimstone tendencies, Gallaudet had a natural affinity for children and an immediate empathy for the languageless deaf girl. His own sickliness had excluded him from the rough-and-tumble play of childhood; he too had been forced to stand apart. He summoned her. That afternoon, he taught her to write the word HAT in the dirt with a stick. Confident that she understood, he discussed her situation with her father. They agreed that Alice could and should be educated. But surely there were others like Alice? Why not start a school?

Most other wealthy parents of deaf children had been content to hire tutors for their own children, period. Dr. Cogswell's concern went beyond the plight of his daughter; he recognized the need for a school to serve all the deaf children of New England. They had a Constitutional right to an education. He shrewdly enlisted the aid of other wealthy citizens, some of whom also had deaf children. He had a census taken by Congregationalist ministers, which showed that there were 84 deaf persons in Connecticut alone—enough to warrant the establishment of a school. Finally, he called together a meeting of ten "city fathers," and Gallaudet was chosen to go to Europe and learn whatever he could about educating the deaf. He accepted eagerly. In just one evening, they raised sufficient funds for him to undertake the journey. The goal: to establish a school for the deaf in Hartford.

Gallaudet was not successful in getting assistance from the Braidwood school. As with other oralists of that time, the Braidwood family guarded their "secret" techniques jealously. They enjoyed a profitable monopoly on education of the deaf in the English-speaking world, and had no intention of giving away their methodology for free. Disgusted and disappointed, Gallaudet went to a public demonstration given by the Abbé Sicard in London. Waiting out the political turmoil then raging in France (he was not on good terms with Napoleon), the abbé was giving public lectures about the French method of educating the deaf and demonstrations of the intellectual abilities of two of his prize pupils, Jean Massieu and Laurent Clerc. The audience was invited to ask them questions—such as definitions of abstract concepts—which the abbé interpreted to the Deaf men in Sign. Taking turns, they wrote their answers, in French, on a large slateboard. These answers were often witty, sometimes profound. Gallaudet was astounded.

Sicard invited Gallaudet to visit the French National Institute. Finally, in 1816, despairing of accomplishing anything in England, Gallaudet embarked for Paris. He was accorded a warm welcome at the Institute.

Even though he was given free access to all the classes, had private tutoring by Sicard and Massieu, and studied diligently, Gallaudet recognized that there was simply not enough time to master everything he needed to know to teach the deaf. Dwindling funds forced him to book passage home. He boldly proposed to Clerc that he accompany him to the States to help set up the new school. (This was not part of the original plan, of course.) Clerc, who had an adventurous streak, agreed. Although Sicard at first refused, he finally relented, agreeing to loan Clerc for 3 years.

During their 51 days on board the *Mary Augusta*, Clerc taught Gallaudet the fine points of FSL, and Gallaudet taught Clerc English. (Clerc became an excellent writer in this second language.)

When Gallaudet and Clerc arrived in the States, they set about raising funds for the school. Gallaudet was a superb orator—and a persuasive one. Alice Cogswell had been placed in a nearby girls' school for the time being, and was barely literate. On arrival in Hartford, Clerc met Cogswell and Alice. There was great joy at their first meeting—the urbane, cultured, and brilliant Parisian gentleman and the child for whose sake he had come. Both deaf. Cogswell must have been mightily reassured. Gallaudet's bold gamble was to pay off— quite handsomely.

The American Asylum for the Instruction of Deaf and Dumb Persons opened in Hartford on April 15, 1817. Alice Cogswell was the first to enroll. Clerc and Gallaudet each taught classes. Sign language was used in class. Clerc used FSL, fingerspelling, and, for a time, the cumbersome "methodical signs" used in the French National Institute classes, but soon found (to his dismay) that his students were "changing" his signs. What they were doing, of course, was adapting them to their preferences. A number of them already had their own way of signing—a background in native Sign, so to speak. Ultimately, Clerc discarded the "methodical signs," and ASL became more and more a distinct language, used inside and outside the classroom, although it really wasn't thought of as *a language* until William Stokoe subjected it to linguistic analysis 143 years later. It was simply called "sign(s)" or "deaf sign." ASL was not taught as a subject in the class; it was employed as the medium of communication, along with written English. The school's goals were English literacy, industriousness, and Congregational-style morality.

The curriculum did *not* include speech training. It was considered unprofitable, a waste of time, as the majority of students would not derive enough benefit from it to make it worthwhile. A few "semi-mutes" (students who had lost their hearing after learning how to talk, or those with a moderate hearing loss) were given some articulation training, but aside from these, there was no attempt to teach speech skills. The emphasis was on education.

Clerc settled down to a busy and productive life in Hartford and largely spent the rest of his life there; he made only three more visits to France. Gallaudet became supervisor of the institution. Underpaid and overworked, he was frequently in conflict with the school board. Both Clerc and Gallaudet married "Hartford" students. In 1818, Clerc married Eliza Crocker Boardman, one of his first pupils. It was the first Deaf marriage in the country. Soon afterwards, Gallaudet married Sophia Fowler, the future "queen of the Deaf community." Both marriages were happy. All the children were hearing, but the eldest and youngest Gallaudet children each continued their father's mission. The younger Thomas Gallaudet established the first Deaf church in the States. Edward Miner Gallaudet was the founder and first president of what is now Gallaudet University. They were native Signers, and most likely learned ASL from their mother.

Two of the first Hartford pupils became teachers of the deaf, initiating an honored American tradition of the best deaf pupils becoming teachers of the deaf themselves. The Hartford Asylum became a model for the establishment of dozens of other schools for the deaf—Fanwood (New York), Pennsylvania, Indiana—all across the country. It also led to the establishment of Gallaudet University—the world's first (and still the only) liberal-arts college for the Deaf.

Within a remarkably short time, ASL-based education led to the formation of a real Deaf community, complete with clubs, churches, organizations, sports, and a flourishing Deaf press, known as the "Little Paper Family." The residential schools created a class of highly-educated, skilled Deaf people who were, in fact, bilingual—fluent in Sign, and articulate in written English. We call this the "Golden Age of Deaf Culture."

In 1850, Gallaudet and Clerc were honored at a convocation of all living Hartford alumni. (Dr. Cogswell and Alice had both died in 1830.) It was a beautiful sight—the reunion of dozens of educated and skilled Deaf citizens, alumni of Hartford. Gallaudet died the next year. Clerc lived long enough to witness the upsurge of oralism that threatened to undo everything he had labored to achieve.

Key to illustrations on page 28

"Mother"

American Sign Language

Australian Sign Language

Spanish Sign Language

Japanese Sign Language

Gestuno
(International Sign Language)

"Man"

"Woman"

Chapter 2

Is there one sign language for all countries?

o more so than there is one spoken language for all countries! But everywhere you find Deaf people, you will find sign language. The impulse to communicate is universal. For deaf people, the impulse to sign is universal. Deaf children not exposed to any standard sign language will invent their own sign systems ("home sign"). Every national sign language, however, is different. In Europe, even within a single country, there can be tremendous variation from city to city, while American Sign Language, although possessing many regional dialects and "accents," is standardized enough to be easily understood by ASL users (an estimated 500,000) from coast to coast. So a Deaf Californian and a Deaf New Englander will have no difficulty understanding each other. ASL is also used in Canada, which extends its scope considerably.

Deaf people in the States were using sign language long before Laurent Clerc, the first Deaf educator in America, arrived from France, bringing French Sign Language with him. It is thought that the native sign language of Chilmark and Tisbury, the Martha's Vineyard communities with an unusually high incidence of hereditary deafness, evolved from Old Kentish Sign Language, as the earliest deaf settlers came from the Kentish region of England.

Although ASL was subsequently influenced by FSL (and thus has some recognizably French signs), many such borrowed signs have been modified over time. But while ASL belongs to the same family as FSL and Spanish Sign Language, which all have some signs in common ("baby," "book"), it is quite different from British Sign Language, which remained largely impervious to French influence. Nonetheless, the French National Institute (where Clerc trained and taught) sent its teachers to several countries, including Holland, Denmark, Spain, and Russia, so FSL left its mark on those sign languages too.

Scandinavian sign languages (e.g., Swedish Sign Language) form an important group, rich and vibrant, whose artistic possibilities have begun to be explored. Asian sign languages (e.g., Japanese Sign Language, Taiwanese Sign Language) differ from any European sign language. Each school for the deaf in Japan—and 11 of the 12 are oral—has its own sign-language system, as used by the students. Some African sign languages are influenced by the native sign languages of missionaries. There are undoubtedly several complete and rich sign languages that have never been adequately studied or recognized.

Every different sign language reflects its own history, culture, and social mores. Thus (in most of these different sign languages) you will find completely different signs for universal concepts: "mother," "father," "boy," "girl," "day," "night," "tree," "water," "good," "bad," and so forth.* Each sign language may have a myriad of regional variations. And what is a perfectly acceptable sign in one language may turn out to be an obscenity in another! E.g., the perfectly innocent sign for "brother" in Taiwanese Sign Language bears an uncanny resemblance to the vulgar "up yours" gesture popularized by hearing (*and* deaf) Americans.

But Signers from one country seem to have less trouble

establishing communication with Signers from another than do their speaking counterparts. Deaf people can be very inventive, even ingenious, in bridging language gaps! They improvise, using gestures, pantomime, expressions—whatever works—until they establish some sort of mutual comprehension, and build on that foundation.

"International sign language" does exist to some extent. An "artificial" international vocabulary, "Gestuno," which functions as a kind of visual Esperanto, was developed in the mid-70s by the Commission on Unification of Signs of the World Federation of the Deaf. Gestuno hasn't really caught on. It *is* useful for international gatherings of Deaf people (e.g., the Gala Opening Performance at The DEAF WAY Conference and Festival in Washington, D.C., July 1989), where it's impractical to throng the stage with dozens of interpreters in everybody's native sign languages. American Deaf performers were specially drilled in Gestuno, and used it to introduce acts and give simple communications to the audience—"Welcome, ladies and gentlemen;" "No smoking, please;" "No flash photography allowed at performances;" "I hope you enjoy our show." The signs used are as simple, logical, and universally recognizable as possible. Since Gestuno was developed by a committee, it's not a real language. But Gestuno was partly based on ASL, which, as the world's most well-known and popular sign language, is the closest thing we have to a "universally" recognized one.

---

*In many spoken languages across the world, the word for *mother* begins with or contains the letter "m." For example: *mater* (Latin); *mama* (Italian); *mère* (French); *maman* (French vernacular); *madre* (Spanish); *maht* (Russian); *matka* (Polish); *Mutter* (German); *mor* (Danish, Swedish, Norwegian); *imma* (Hebrew).

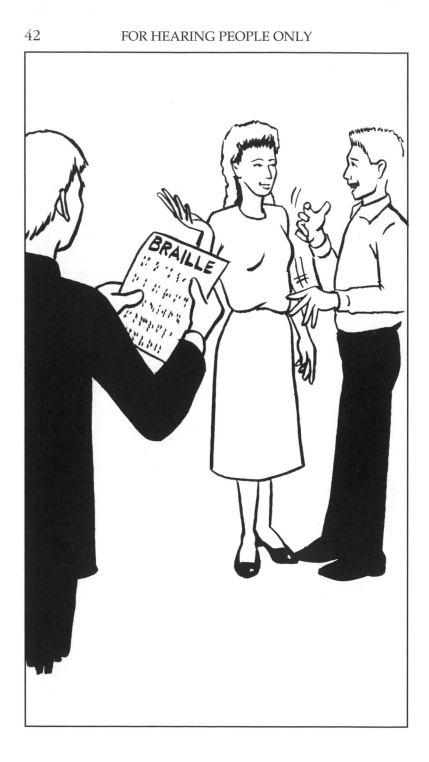

Chapter 3

Is there any similarity between Braille and ASL?

one whatever, but you'd be surprised how many folks apparently think they're the same thing. Some hearing people have told us that when they first saw Deaf people signing to each other, they immediately thought, "Oh, they're using Braille. They must be blind!" Why?

Blind people are visible to us in a way that the Deaf aren't. Many blind people use special white canes; some also have guide dogs with distinctive harnesses. A blind person waiting to cross a traffic-congested street or boarding a city bus is immediately recognized as blind and quickly offered assistance—an arm while crossing the street, a front seat on the bus. (A very general statement, this.)

Deaf people, however, are not immediately recognizable as "Deaf." There will be no telltale cane or (in most cases) dog, no dark glasses, nothing out of the ordinary except, perhaps, one or two hearing aids, if they're visible at all. Thus, hearing people undoubtedly have very clear images of what blind people "look like," but no clear notion of how Deaf people "look." Not until Deaf people are seen communicating with each other in Sign (or a hearing stranger approaches, mumbles something to them, and gets no response or a gesture of incomprehension) are they identifiable as "Deaf."

In our culture, blindness has garnered more recognition and respect than deafness. We suspect that far more hearing schoolchildren know about Louis Braille than about Laurent Clerc. They may also have a clearer notion of Braille, a tactile code, than ASL, a visual language. Consequently, when they see native Signers for the first time (and this is our wild guess), they associate signing with the language of the blind, not the language of the Deaf. Or they assume that most Deaf people "know Braille."

Just for the record, Braille is not a language like ASL. It's a code, a way of translating "flat copy"—written and printed media—into a tactile form: raised dots in a matrix pattern read with the fingertips. Not all blind people read Braille (and it is by no means the only available code, or the easiest to learn). Many blind people find it indispensable, and a good number use Braille books, typewriters, notetaker punches, Telebraille machines, and Braille-printing computers with voice synthesizers, like the state-of-the-art Kurzweil Personal Reader. Braille has much more in common with Morse Code than with ASL. But Morse Code, unlike Braille, *can* be used to communicate directly with blind people (i.e., conversationally), by substituting taps and strokes for dots and dashes. It is thus—*very* roughly—equivalent to fingerspelling.*

Deaf-blind people do use tactile signing and fingerspelling (either done directly in the palm, or in the usual front-of-body position and "read" with the fingertips) to converse with each other or with sighted Deaf people. They are extraordinarily adept at it. Blind hearing people (especially those who have attended combined schools for the deaf and blind) may be skilled in this as well; fingerspelling is relatively easy to learn. But you will never see two people standing on the corner having a conversation "in Braille."

*Interestingly, Samuel F.B. Morse had a deaf wife, and communicated with her by "tapping out Morse code in her hands!" See Harlan Lane, **When the Mind Hears**, p. 276.

Chapter 4

Wasn't French Sign Language invented by the Abbé de l'Epée?

o. French Sign Language was invented by Deaf people. It was the exclusive property of the French deaf community, for there were a fairly large number of deaf people living in Paris in the 18th century. They may have been forced to the outer fringes of society, but they had the rudiments of a recognizable Deaf culture—namely, a language.

The Abbé Charles-Michel de l'Epée (1712-1789) was a "neighborhood priest" whose involvement with deaf people began in the mid-1700s when he met twin deaf sisters whose mother begged him to teach them. (Another priest, the Abbé Simon Vanin, had been working with them, teaching them moral concepts by means of pictures of the saints, but had died.) Accordingly, l'Epée sought to instruct them. His original purpose was, of course, religious as well as humanitarian. He wanted to save deaf people's souls from damnation. In order to achieve salvation, deaf people had to understand the sacraments. They had to have access to education. But the Abbé had to communicate with the deaf.

He researched what available information there was on deaf education, and adapted the Spanish system of fingerspelling. More important, he was the first hearing person to go to the deaf community, to learn its language, to let deaf people teach *him*. Ultimately, he founded the first successful school for deaf students in Paris, which became the National Institute for Deaf-Mutes. In his classes, he used signs from FSL with an added set of signs he *had* invented, *les signes méthodiques* ("methodical signs") which represented aspects of French grammar that lacked equivalents in FSL. Erroneously, he assumed that FSL lacked grammatical structure, and wished to remedy this supposed deficiency. The Abbé's "methodical signs" were something of an early "Signed French" system. They were ugly and cumbersome, and his successors modified them—and later dropped them altogether. But the students used "pure" FSL in the dormitories—and so French Deaf culture began in earnest.

Previous educators of the deaf had imposed their sometimes ridiculous ideas, misguided philosophies, and erroneous notions about language onto their pupils and never took into account the fact that deaf people already had a highly-developed *visual* means of communication. All the oralists tried to make their deaf pupils function as hearing persons. They all failed to do so. The Abbé de l'Epée approached deaf people with a more open mind. To paraphrase Harlan Lane's monumental history, **When the Mind Hears**, the Abbé was the first known educator who bothered to learn from the deaf themselves, and that is why, for all his own mistaken notions, he is remembered as a friend of deaf people.*

The Abbé had nothing to do with the invention of sign language. Rather, he *recognized* the importance of sign language as the best way to communicate with and educate deaf people. And he *pioneered* its use in an institutional setting.

L'Epée's successor, the Abbé Roch-Ambroise Cucurron Sicard (1742-1822), wrote a two-volume treatise on deaf education, **Théorie des Signes** (1808). This book found its way into Dr. Mason Cogswell's library; Dr. Cogswell gave it to Thomas Hopkins Gallaudet, who had just met

9-year-old Alice Cogswell. Gallaudet studied it and ultimately adapted it for American use. During his sojourn in London, he met Sicard, and went to the National Institute in Paris to learn the method firsthand. The French approach—the use of the native sign language to teach the native written language—was known as the "silent" or "natural" method. In contrast to the oralists of that time, its proponents made no secret of it; they disseminated it, demonstrated it publicly, shared it with whomever wished to learn it, and trained teachers to establish free public schools for the deaf throughout Europe, including Russia. This French model in turn inspired the American model.

Sicard, who directed the Institute during and after the French Revolution, had a remarkable pupil, Jean Massieu, an erstwhile shepherd who became one of the first truly educated Deaf persons. And Massieu's pupil was the legendary Laurent Clerc, the first teacher of the deaf in the United States. Clerc brought FSL to the States, and to this day, American Sign Language shows a distinct "French" influence.

*"Still, it was the abbé de l'Epée, son of the king's architect, who first turned to the poor, despised, illiterate deaf and said, 'Teach me,' And this act of humility gained him everlasting glory. It is his true title to our gratitude, for in becoming the student of his pupils, in seeking to learn their signs, he equipped himself to educate them and to found the education of the deaf. For this reason, the deaf everywhere have always excused him for failing to see that the sign language of the French deaf community was a complete language in its own right, not merely a collection of signs, and did not need to be made to 'conform to clear rules'—French word order and word endings, to be transformed into 'manual French'—in order to serve as the vehicle for instructing the deaf."
—Harlan Lane (writing as Laurent Clerc), **When the Mind Hears**, p. 63.

Chapter 5

"Can you explain the sentence structure of ASL? Is it a result of its French background?"

I am presently enrolled at Gallaudet University in their beginning ASL course. Do you have or know of a text which can explain the sentence structure of ASL? I assume it's a result of its French background. At Gallaudet we haven't gotten into that as yet; we've been concentrating on gestures and signs for basics like numbers, colors, living quarters, alphabet, and shapes. I realize gestures play a major role in the language, but I've also noticed that questions are not in an English order.

R. M.
Wheaton, Maryland

he syntactical structure of ASL is not really due to a French origin. Yes, ASL *was* deeply influenced and enriched by FSL. The French influence is most evident in its vocabulary—some 60% of its signs are borrowed from FSL. But ASL originated in the United States. In its oldest form, it existed well over a century before Laurent Clerc brought FSL to the States in 1817. Its syntax is peculiarly "American," and is logically "the way it is" because it's a true visual/spatial/gestural language—perfectly adapted to the needs of Deaf Americans who communicate visually. It owes nothing to English.[1]

Crudely speaking, in English you have a fairly pat

syntactical structure—modifier-subject-verb-object (MSVO). Other combinations—SMVO, MSVO, SVOM— are also possible. But ASL has a syntactical flexibility you won't find in English. The word order varies according to the emphasis—and the nuances of expression—a sort of visual-kinetic-poetic license which adds vividness to the simplest statement.[2] English is dry, sequential. In ASL the entire body is used expressively to convey information. Spoken English uses a string of phonemes (sounds), words, and sentences. Period. ASL can expand the expression of each sign according to the signer's mood, feelings, or attitude. English cannot do that; it's much more limited. The expressive possibilities of ASL are virtually limitless. English is uni-dimensional; ASL multi-dimensional.

In ASL, information about nouns, subject, or object, is incorporated into directional verbs. Verbs are inflected in a way foreign to English. There are features like classifiers, which are lacking in English. (Classifiers are also found in Navajo, a highly visual spoken language which, until recently, lacked a written form. ASL and Navajo use classifiers in the exact same way; their morphology [word formation] is similar. ASL is thus structurally closer to Navajo than to English![3]) And the face is used as a grammatical marker—as with questions and negatives. These are but a few aspects which make assimilation of ASL difficult even for motivated hearing people.

This is also why innumerable Manually Coded English (MCE) systems have been devised—to make it easier for native English speakers (hearing teachers) to teach English to native ASL users (i.e., deaf children). The vocabulary of signs is borrowed, adapted—or butchered—from ASL, but the syntax imposed on the signs is that of English. Hearing people taking beginning sign-language classes usually learn Signed English. Likewise, Deaf people tend to use a rough-and-ready variation, Pidgin Sign English (PSE), when communicating with hearing people—a signed form of English is easier for the hearing people to understand. Neither MCE nor PSE are true languages. They are signed forms of communication. With ASL you have to abandon "English thinking" and think **visually**. It's not easy.

Here are a few texts that can help explain the structure of ASL (see also Bibliography):

William C. Stokoe, **Sign Language Structure**, 1960; rpt., Silver Spring, Md: Linstok Press.

William C. Stokoe, Dorothy C. Casterline, and Carl G. Croneberg, **A Dictionary of American Sign Language on Linguistic Principles**. Illus. 1965; rev. ed., Silver Spring, Md: Linstok Press, 1976.

Ronnie Wilbur, **American Sign Language: Linguistic and Applied Dimensions**. Boston: Little, Brown, 1987.

Sherman Wilcox and Phyllis Wilcox, **Learning to See: American Sign Language as a Second Language**. Educational Resources Information Center/Center for Applied Linguistics/Prentice Hall Regents, 1991.

[1] Can a native ASL user understand a native FSL user? The answer is yes—given time to familiarize each other. Understanding doesn't come immediately, but there is *some* common linguistic ground.

[2] ASL certainly has grammatical rules. But it isn't accurate to say that the subject always comes first, or even "usually" or "often." The subject may be implied or dropped. What is true of ASL is not necessarily true of other sign languages; there is no universal parallel structure.

[3] If not for Navajo, we might still be waiting for linguistic recognition of ASL. Navajo is a spoken language used by hearing people—and yet it has classifiers, just as ASL does. Navajo established a precedent for recognizing ASL as a full-fledged language. We are fortunate in that Navajo, as a native language, survived at all. Most other (Native) American Indian languages have vanished without being recorded.

Chapter 6

Is ASL a written language? (And can it be translated into written English?)

ince American Sign Language (ASL) is a purely visual/gestural language, it has no written form. (Only a relatively small percentage of spoken languages have written forms, for that matter.) Authors of ASL dictionaries and textbooks are therefore faced with the problem of "reproducing" in print a language that "cannot be written down"! As the introduction to Dennis Cokely and Charlotte Baker's first ASL textbook puts it:

> ASL is not a written language. This means that there are no newspapers, magazines, books, etc., written in ASL. Because ASL does not have a written form, we generally have to use English to write about ASL. This means using English words (called "glosses") when trying to translate the meaning of ASL signs and for trying to write down ASL sentences. [1]

Dr. William C. Stokoe, the pioneering researcher of ASL who did so much to gain linguistic respect for ASL as a distinct and living language, published the first ASL dictionary in 1965, for which he devised a set of very useful linguistic Sign symbols, showing at a glance the five parameters of each Sign: handshape, palm orientation, location, movement, and repetition. Cokely and Baker's pioneering ASL textbooks (1980) utilize a "code" of symbols and abbreviations. As these books emphasize, the English words used to translate the meaning of the ASL sentences are an approximation—"glosses."

Valerie Sutton published a bilingual newspaper, **The Sign Writer**, using an ASL-based pictographic code (stylized signs, movements, and facial grammar), the most ambitious attempt we've seen so far. There are a number of computer programs, and much experimental work is being done in this field. But as far as rendering ASL in written form in a print medium, there are considerable difficulties.

Even a good ASL dictionary—and there are some very attractive ones on the mass market for non-scholars—acknowledges its limitations. Although it will clearly illustrate a good number of common signs (with arrows and blur-lines to indicate movement or repetition), in reality, the gloss accompanying the illustration may depict only one possible meaning of the sign. ASL's vocabulary does not correspond to that of English, and its grammatical structure is quite different. One of the things that makes ASL so fascinating (and difficult to learn from scratch) is its subtlety. You can't get that from a dictionary; you have to experience it firsthand with skilled signers. Second best is a series of good videotapes or films—a visual medium.

ASL is not a written language. In everyday usage, it is never written. It can, of course, be coded, glossed, or translated into English. But the gloss or text will only be an approximation of the ASL. Grammatically correct ASL can be rendered in grammatically correct English, but it loses something in translation—which is, of course, a universal problem.[2]

---

[1] Dennis Cokely and Charlotte Baker, **American Sign Language: a student text** (Units 1-9),"Note To the Student," x.

[2] Consider the title of Marcel Proust's **À la recherche du temps perdu**. It is generally translated as **Remembrance of Things Past**—a phrase taken from Shakespeare's Sonnet 30—but a closer translation would be **In Search of Lost Time**. The opening sentence of the

first volume, **Du côté de chez Swann (Swann's Way)**, reads in the original French: "Longtemps, je me suis couché de bonne heure." C.K. Scott Moncrieff's standard translation reads: "For a long time, I used to go to bed early." What gets lost is Proust's music—the languid cadence, the rhythm of the long, solemn vowels and consonants. The original is poetic; the translation is banal.

Chapter 7

How do deaf people learn sign language?

hey learn it from each other. Until recently, American Sign Language was never formally taught to deaf children; the only ASL classes available were, ironically, for hearing college students. (With the advent of the Bilingual-Bicultural approach to deaf education, and recognition of ASL as a foreign language by a number of states, the situation is changing. Slowly.) From the beginning, deaf children who have deaf parents have always taught the other deaf kids ASL at residential schools. As Arden Neisser observes:

[F]or close to a century, [sign language] was matter-of-factly ignored, despised and outlawed, neither taught nor tolerated in classrooms for the deaf. Teachers in the schools were completely unfamiliar with it, did not use it, and could not understand it. They were trained in oral methods... (...) Oral programs begin by teaching the children to make sounds, then words, one at a time. Deaf children who have been in oral kindergarten programs have learned, by age five, perhaps fifty words. At the same time, a child with normal hearing has a vocabulary of several thousand words; and a deaf child of deaf parents who has learned ASL as a first language has a vocabulary of several thousand signs. But most deaf children (around 90 percent) have hearing parents and enter school with no ASL and such a restricted knowledge of English that they are virtually without any functioning language at all. (...)

It is estimated that 90 percent of deaf adults who were deaf as children use ASL, and most of them learned it at schools for the deaf—from each other. They simply signed behind their teachers' backs.[1] (...) ASL is said to be the only language in the world that is transmitted from child to child.[2]

Deaf children, arriving at school, are plunged into an ASL environment in the playgrounds, cafeteria, and (especially) the dormitories. Even if signing is forbidden in class (e.g., Clarke School) or if signed-English-only is used there, deaf kids use ASL everywhere *outside* the classroom; they're surrounded by it. New kids pick it up quickly. Within a few months, they've become skillful signers, ASL their first language. When they grow up, many alumni marry another deaf person, a veteran ASL user. Most deaf parents (an estimated 90%) have hearing children. The 10% who have deaf children usually send them to the residential schools, where they teach the other kids ASL. Thus ASL has been transmitted from generation to generation.

Some deaf persons learn ASL later in life—on arrival at NTID, for example.[3] But the best way to become proficient in ASL is to achieve total immersion in it—living with Deaf people—or, second best, through everyday social contact with native ASL users. Third best is to associate with them regularly in the classroom or office.

It's certainly possible to learn ASL as an adult. Some late-deafened adults do so, enthusiastically, and do well. But it takes time, commitment, practice, good teachers, and the right attitude. (What worthwhile venture doesn't?) A real "amateur" attitude is to pant, "I want to become fluent overnight!" or sigh, "I'll never learn all this!"

Taking a course in "Basic Sign" is OK for starters, but not all sign-language classes are created equal! Videotapes of skilled native ASL users are good as a supplement, but real live person-to-person interaction is the best way—as all deaf kids know. There's just no substitute.

[1] Arden Neisser, **The Other Side of Silence: Sign Language and the Deaf Community in America** , p. 8.

[2] Neisser, p. 47.

[3] The National Technical Institute for the Deaf (NTID) is one of 8 colleges of Rochester Institute of Technology in Rochester, New York. It attracts deaf students from a wide variety of backgrounds— oral, ASL/Signing, mainstreamed, and residential. (See Chapter 46.)

Chapter 8

Can people who are deaf from birth appreciate jokes and puns that involve homonyms (sound-alike words)?

Here are a few examples of homonym
(phonetic) humor:

Mini-skirt: wearing a peril. (Robert Kuranz)

**Q. Why can't a bicycle stand by itself?
A: Because it's two-tired.**

**As one horse said to the other:
"I can't remember your mane, but your pace is familiar."**

**Q: What's round and purple and conquered the world?
A: Alexander the Grape.**

 okes like these which rely on homonyms (or puns, for that matter) are pretty much incomprehensible to many born-deaf people. To enjoy English wordplay, you really need some degree of everyday immersion in English as a spoken language, *or* a top-notch bilingual education. Young hearing children love wordplay (the sillier the better), but then, a normal hearing 6-year-old already has a vocabulary of some 3,000 words and intuitively constructs grammatically-correct sentences. A child born deaf grows up without that unconscious absorption of spoken English that all hearing English-speaking people take for granted. Far too many deaf children receive a strictly inferior education. They often start school without *any* real language at all! As a result, their English vocabulary tends to be quite limited and augmented slowly and painfully; English skills "halt" at about a third- to fifth-grade level. Most congenitally deaf people can't be expected to understand the whimsical aspects of English wordplay, much less enjoy it. Consequently, much English humor, even if it's written, is "oral-based" and not accessible to them. It excludes them. So, no, they would not appreciate this kind of humor at all.

Real Deaf humor is visually based. It encompasses mime, gesture, cinematic effects (like zooming, close-ups, fast and slow motion), and a lot of spontaneous sign-play. Although hearing people without prior exposure to ASL can enjoy the beauty and cartoon-like wit of Signing, much of it is as incomprehensible to them as "Hearing" humor is to those born deaf. You really need a strong background in ASL to begin to appreciate the nuances and whimsy of Deaf humor.

As for translating English puns and phonetic wordplay into Sign or fingerspelling, it doesn't work very well. Humor is an "in-cultural" attribute, and it translates badly. As that proverb about analyzing humor goes, it's like dissecting a frog—you can take it apart to see how it works, but it dies in the process.

A slight digression

A response to the original installment:
I take issue with the conclusions [here].

I also take issue with the implications in the title "For Hearing People Only." Let's stop referring to "hearing people" as though they be a superior group of human beings on a higher plane. (I don't mean British Airways or American Airlines, ha ha! Geddit? Higher plane? Oh, well, I was only trying to be plain-ly punny.) Let's refer to hearing people, especially those who have inept hands in Deafness, for what most of them really are: non-Deaf. They have no inkling of what we Deaf people are, want, need, and can do. Their only concern is to un-Deaf us as much as possible.

They are the people responsible for the situation [you] describe so aptly: "Far too many Deaf children receive a strictly inferior education. . . . [And] English skills 'halt' at about a third- to fifth-grade level."

It is this "strictly inferior education" (applying to non-Deaf as well as Deaf children) which accounts for anyone (Deaf or non-Deaf) being unable to appreciate puns and other English word-play.

The first two examples of 'homonym' (phonetic) humor involve not just an awareness of sound but also of pronunciation and spelling. The second two examples have nothing at all to do with homonyms (or homographs, or, what [the reader asking the question] really means, homophones), or phonetics, for that matter. They have to do with a person's stock of words and common phrases, spelling skills, historical-cultural knowledge—and ability to read and write and play with and enjoy words, whether English or ASL.

Being Deaf, Percy (Oh, I know Percy's not your name; I was just punning *per se*) has nothing to do with understanding English or ASL or any language.

David Anthony
Boulder, CO
(True self born Deaf and mother father both true self self born Deaf;
English tease tease like, and English teach teach like.)

Our reply:
Arguing about terminology is tricky. We titled the feature "For Hearing People Only" not out of deference to their "superiority," but because so many hearing people are pathetically under-informed, misinformed, or, on the brighter side, curious about Deaf people. We thought they warranted a special feature where they could share their questions and get straight answers elucidating different aspects of Deaf culture.

True, many hearing people feel that "aurally-handicapped" or "hearing-impaired" is a more apt term for us. But they're not *our* terms. We didn't title our magazine "**HEARING-IMPAIRED LIFE.**"

—Letters to the Editor, **DEAF LIFE**, April 1990

Chapter 9

Are there such things as accents among signers from different areas of the country or world?

ndeed there are! One fascinating aspect of sign language is that every signer signs differently, developing his or her own unique style. Some sign abruptly, angularly; some sloppily, some gracefully. Some sign "small," some "large" and clear. Just as with spoken languages: everyone enunciates a bit differently, and there will be a great difference in quality between the voice of a trained performing artist and that of someone who slurs, mumbles, and has sloppy articulation. Instead of vocal accents, signers have visual/gestural accents.

Conversely, every sign-language system "works" differently. Thai Sign Language (from our observation) looks very formal; the face has a tighter, more deadpan look. British Sign Language (BSL) might, at first glance, be mistaken for American Sign Language, but it "moves" completely differently. A native user of BSL who learned ASL would undoubtedly retain a BSL intonation or "accent."

In the past, even within the boundaries of one European country, signers from one city might not understand signers from a different city. But in the United States, ASL has achieved a remarkable level of homogeneity. Native signers from one area can easily understand those from a distant area. However, as with spoken American English, there are many regional variations, with some signs peculiar to a specific area or community (such as Deaf Blacks in Georgia). There are several different "regional" signs for "Halloween," "Christmas," "birthday," and "outside." (It's especially true with sexual signs.) You can't necessarily guess right off what part of the country a signer is from, but the variations can be (and have been) pinpointed, mapped, and studied. And, yes, there is such a thing as Sign dialect humor. A skilled storyteller can make effective use of comic "hillbilly" sign, pompous "Oxford English," or hip "jive talk."

There will be differences between the ASL usage of a college graduate and a relatively uneducated grassroots-Deaf person. We have white-collar and blue-collar ASL. As in any culture, such differences can be used as weapons of oppression. Snobbery certainly exists in the Deaf community. Those who are proud of the purity of their ASL, those who enjoy showing off their advanced "Englishy" vocabulary (with lots of big fingerspelled words), and those who have learned ASL relatively late in life—all have very different accents, and each may look down on the others. The choice of codes—ASL or a form of signed English—has immense political and social implications. Until recently, Sign English was considered correct, educated, "high-class," and ASL "low-class." This is the satiric crux of Gil Eastman's pioneering ASL play, *Sign Me Alice,* a very funny take-off on Shaw's *Pygmalion.*

Deaf people do tease each other lightheartedly about their accents. There are bilingual hearing people—primarily those with Deaf parents—whose ASL accent is "pure." Since relatively few hearing people become fluent signers, a native signer can usually (though not invariably) recognize a hearing person by the slightly halting quality of their signing and the way they use their face and body: "Oh, you sign with a Hearing accent!"

A few American regional Sign variations.
Top row: *birthday*; center row: *soon*; bottom row: *outside*.

Alabama

California

Maine,
Massachusetts,
Pennsylvania

California, Florida,
Illinois, Missouri

Maine, Utah,
Washington

New York

Arkansas, Kentucky,
Wisconsin

Massachusetts,
Pennsylvania

Michigan,
New York

Chapter 10

"I want to learn bigger signs."

Just recently I went to cheerleading camp. There I met four deaf girls. They were the only thing that made me want to stay at camp longer. It was very interesting to my friend and I. Even though they couldn't hear, they were the funnest people to be with.

The reason I'm writing is because I'm really interested in how to talk sign language in bigger signs so if I see them I'll be able to talk to them. It's very important to me. I was watching a show the other day and a little deaf kid got lost and everybody was trying to talk to him in words; they had no idea he was deaf until someone came along who knows sign language. If I see someone like that who needs help, I want to be able to help them. Sign language is something I would never take for granted. I want to know if there's anything you can send me that will help me learn bigger signs.

T. K.
Fairfax, Missouri

The best place to start is your local public library. Ask the reference librarian where you can find materials relating to sign language, and resources on deafness and media. The library should have at least a few helpful books you can check out. And if you can't find anything, you can have the librarian contact another library to get it for you. The library may also be able to point you towards local resources, such as sign-language classes, Deaf clubs, or organizations.

As for making the signs bigger, all you need to remember is that the normal "signing space" extends from the top of the head to the waist, and from shoulder to shoulder. When communicating with another deaf person, make sure to give them enough space to sign freely *and* to get a clear view of your signs. Signers tend to stand a bit further away from each other than hearing people do while talking. A comfortable distance—at least an extended arm's length—ensures good readability. Ask those you're signing to. They'll show you.

The important thing is to get into practice, and, if possible, find someone who's skillful in signing to practice with. That makes it more fun.

Signing space: the upper torso and head

Deaf Awareness 5-Minute Quiz

Chapters 1—10

Answers are on the bottom of the page, upside down.

True or False:

1. American Sign Language is quite similar to British Sign Language. just as spoken American English is very close to British English.

2. The Abbé de l'Epée was the first educator who recognized that sign language was the natural language of the deaf, but thought that it was a collection of signs without grammatical structure.

3. All sign languages have the same basic structure—the subject comes first.

4. Various writing systems have been developed for ASL, but outside of textbooks, none are in very wide use.

5. Deaf children usually learn sign language from each other.

Chapter 11

"I know it takes a great deal of practice, but do you have any information on how to better accomplish fingerspelling?"

In the first [ASL] class I took, we learned fingerspelling. However, I am having trouble "reading" fingerspelling from another speller. My speed is also slow. I know it takes a great deal of practice, but do you have any information on how to better accomplish this?

R.M.
Wheaton, Maryland

ingerspelling is a vital kinetic-visual skill, an essential component of sign-language communication.* A basic knowledge of fingerspelling will take you a long way, as you can fingerspell any word you don't yet know the correct sign for (or have forgotten, or just aren't sure about). As each handshape corresponds to a specific letter of the alphabet, it's not particularly difficult to learn. Some adult beginners master fingerspelling in a couple of hours or less; others never seem to get the hang of it. Motivation is as important as dexterity. Clarity is more important than speed. It's important to know how to form your letters correctly and clearly, keep your fingers from kinking, maintain a smooth flow, and stay in practice. This, of course, takes time and dedication. Jerkiness, bouncing, and staring at the hands in self-conscious dismay are dead giveaways for the amateur klutz!

We assume you've learned the basics and know the difference between K and P. Setting aside a half-hour every day for practice (if you're a punctilious sort) is ideal. But you can use any duration of "captive time" (such as a bus or taxi ride, solo waiting, watching a boring TV program or a string of commercials) to run through the alphabet a few times. You can take a favorite poem or brief prose item and see if you can fingerspell it clearly. And then there's mirror-practice . . .

Most sign-language textbooks start with fingerspelling exercises. We found a promising oversize booklet in the Rochester Public Library: **Expressive and Receptive Fingerspelling for Adults** by LaVera M. Guillory (Baton Rouge: Claitor's Bookstore, Publishing Div., 1966). The Library of Congress number is 66-17803. The Dewey call number is (q or Oversize) 371.912 G961e (or similar). If you want to go whole hog, you can buy self-instructional videotapes. DawnSignPress, for example, has a 2-hour videotape, *Fingerspelling: Expressive & Receptive Fluency*, which includes an instructional booklet with practice suggestions.

As always, the best advice is to get real-life practice. If you have any friends who are native ASL users, and who are very patient, go for it! Ask them to drill you on expressive and receptive spelling. (And cherish them.) Native ASL users fingerspell at a characteristically "lightning" pace. Yes, it's possible for an adult beginner to achieve great fluency in fingerspelling. You have to train your eyes to "see quickly," just as you have to train your hands to coordinate.

*It should be noted that native Signers do not use very much fingerspelling. They employ it sparingly—for new words, names, and spellings they're unsure of. Fingerspelling is simply the manual representation of English letters; it is NOT sign language. It was long used as an oral teaching aid—to help deaf children recognize and articulate spoken words properly.

Many adults who learn Sign start with fingerspelling. Even if fingerspelling is all you learn, it's a good skill to have. *Everyone* should know how to fingerspell.

Chapter 12

"Are there any home correspondence courses in Basic Sign?"

Dear Sir, Madam:
Received your article for "hearing people only" and like to have more information about deaf people and their culture. Because of injury received in WW II I slowly lose my hearing (nerve damage). I take sign language at Bakersfield College but so far total confusion because of different teaching of same words and different signing of same words. I live rural area in California and it is hard to find deaf persons to talk or sign to. Are there any home correspondence course? because colleges are total concentrated on grades. All I want to learn simple signs if you meet a deaf person every day talk. What are Pidgin Sign English?? I am grateful for any information you can give me.
Thank you so much in advance.

T.S., Lebec, California

 SL is, of course, best learned in company with a fluent Signer. So what to do if you're geographically isolated? We don't know of a "home correspondence course" in Basic Sign, but home videocourses in Basic Sign, ASL, and Sign literature are available from media companies such as Sign Enhancers, DawnSignPress, Sign Media, and DeBee Communications. One advantage of instructional videos is that you can go at your own pace in relaxed surroundings—your own living room. The major disadvantage is that videotapes are costly and you can't browse around before you buy. What's good for one student may not be good for another.

If you don't have access to a VCR, there are some good and enjoyable books on the market. Still, you need face-to-face practice to make sure that you're forming the signs correctly. (We've watched hearing children and adults teaching themselves signs from illustrations. They usually got it wrong.)

Evidently, you've had considerable difficulty because you've picked up a number of different signs for the same word or concept. Many Deaf people use "regional" signs—their signs will vary according to where they're from and which school they attended. Different teachers favor different signs. For adults learning to sign for the first time, some confusion is unavoidable. Even common signs like "what" and "yesterday" may have several variants. They're equally acceptable, but one form (different from the ones you already learned) may be more prevalent in your signing community. What you can do is keep track of the variations you run into. You can make your own flashcards or a chart in your notebook with descriptions, diagrams, or coded sketches. (Or have a friend help you design them.)

As for community resources: Since you live in California, you can contact a local GLAD (Greater Los Angeles Council on Deafness) or DCARA (Deafness, Counseling, Advocacy, and Referral Agency) in San Leandro, and ask the folks there for more information or advice on just which material would be best for you. GLAD's bookstore has a variety of texts and self-study materials like flashcards and videotapes.

Note, too, that several community colleges and agencies offer beginners' Sign classes in a "non-competitive" atmosphere. Many people who take such classes are deafened adults or friends of deaf people. And ALDA (the Association of Late-Deafened Adults) can provide you with support and networking.

(See Chapter 13 for a response to the question on Pidgin Sign English.)

"I am going to the store."

Signed Exact English

I · AM · GO-ING · TO · THE · STORE.

Pidgin Sign English

I · AM · GO · TO · T-H-E · STORE.

American Sign Language

STORE · THAT ONE · I · GO · NOW

Chapter 13

What is Pidgin Sign English?

ere we go again—another labeling problem! Roughly speaking, PSE is an impromptu blend of American Sign Language and English. It's commonly used when ASL-Deaf people communicate with hearing (or deaf) people who are not fluent in ASL, but who do know some signs and fingerspelling. PSE enables native ASL Signers and native English speakers to comfortably communicate with each other.

The syntax (grammatical structure) of ASL is *very* different from that of English. They are two distinct languages. English is primarily an oral/aural (spoken) language; ASL is visual/gestural/spatial. Since they "work" in completely opposite ways, you can see the difficulty of blending the two.

However, signers are an ingenious lot. Because so many hearing people—native English speakers, that is—are unfamiliar with ASL and have difficulty with its "foreign" syntax, signers have "bridged the gap" between English and ASL by employing a sign system that is neither pure ASL nor pure English, but which borrows and modifies elements from both languages. Pidgin Sign English, in other words, is a method of communication—not a *language* as such—which uses signs borrowed from ASL in a basically English word order, but with some grammatical characteristics of ASL. PSE denotes a naturally-developed sign system, as distinct from invented or "artificial" systems of Manually Coded English. (Keeping track of these labels is tricky business. Other terms for PSE are "Sign English," "Ameslish," and "Siglish," depending on whether you're describing non-English signing or non-ASL signing. Confusing? In practice, it's fairly simple. Whatever works, works.)

It should be noted, however, that PSE is *not* the same as Signed English. PSE omits some English grammar and words, and has more "pure ASL" signs in it. But it is not ASL, either. (Remember, it is not a distinct language at all, just a form of signing that borrows from ASL and English.) Particles such as *a* and *the* are commonly omitted, but forms of the verb *to be* are retained. PSE uses more fingerspelling than ASL, but less than Signed English.

Because PSE uses signs in an English word order, it's possible to speak and sign at the same time. It's an adaptable, flexible, and widely-used approach. Chances are, when you see a Sign interpreter in class or "covering" a public event, or see a Deaf person chatting with a hearing friend, they're using PSE. Since ASL is an extraordinarily flexible language, ASL users readily understand signers who use Signed English or PSE— provided that the signing is clear.

When Deaf people communicate with people (hearing *or* deaf) who aren't fluent in ASL, they tend to "switch codes" to Signed English or PSE, which are more readily understandable by native English users as they conform fairly closely to the grammatical structure of English. Hearing people rarely get to see "pure" ASL being used. What they take for ASL may actually be PSE.

How does one recognize PSE? Here's a very simple example. In PSE you would say, "My name is T-H-E-O-D-O-R-A." You would be using the standard ASL signs for "my" and "name," in an English word order. The sign for "is" would be the same as the sign for "true," not the initialized version (which is Signed English). In ASL you would say, "My name T-H-E-O-D-O-R-A."

The word "pidgin," by the way (which has nothing to do with birds), is a corruption of the word "business." **The American Heritage Dictionary** defines it as: "A simplified form of speech, usually a mixture of two or more languages, that has a rudimentary grammar and vocabulary and is used for communication between groups speaking different languages." The term came from "pidgin English," a corruption of "business English."

Chapter 14

"How do I know if someone is using ASL or signed English?"

How do I know if someone is using ASL or signed English? I have some sign language skills which I have learned from family members who are deaf but just recently I learned that there is a difference. I always thought it was just one language, that is, sign language. So I am wondering if you would inform me a little bit more about ASL, maybe some rules or some examples if possible.

S.M.
Sydney, Nova Scotia

hen sign-language students talk about all the different kinds of sign systems, Manually Coded English systems, and variations thereof, they use the term "continuum." What's a sign-language continuum, anyway? It's a diagram representing the entire population of sign-language users—from the purest Signing-Exact-English approach to the purest ASL approach, and all possible blends or variations in between. Think of a broad arc. On the right are the "pure ASL" users; on the left, the "pure English" users. Pidgin Sign English, which borrows features from both ASL and English, would be situated in the middle of the arc, a bit towards the right. Signed English would be a bit more towards the left. But both are distinct from ASL.

As we've already noted, English and ASL are two *very*

distinct languages. One is orally/aurally based; the other is visual/gestural/spatial. It's possible to transpose any English sentence into a visual/gestural/spatial equivalent—at the crudest level, it can be done with fingerspelling, which simply shows each letter as a different handshape—a manual code. It is considerably more difficult to render ASL into spoken or written English. Every time it gets translated, it loses something. When you say "signing," it can be a basic manual rendition of English, or it can be true ASL. There are many shades of possibilities—and many opportunities for confusion as well.

How do you tell ASL from Signed English on sight? Very roughly speaking, you have to catch the rhythm of the signing. ASL has a different flow, a different "look" from Signed English. The rhythm is entirely different because the syntax (sentence structure) of ASL is so different from Signed English. In ASL you would sign "YOU BUY CAR MAYBE YOU?" or "CAR BUY YOU MAYBE?" or "YOU—CAR BUY MAYBE?" (depending on your emphasis and signing style), while using the facial-grammatical question marker, the eyebrow raise/brow crease, and a subtle tilting forward of the head. In Signed English or Pidgin Sign English you'd sign something like "WILL YOU BUY CAR, MAYBE?" with more mouthing of the English words.

To someone not familiar with the language, an ASL conversation looks like a lightning-quick, intense "pantomime" of sorts. ASL is very expressive, eruptive. Since the face is used as a grammatical marker, expressions are "exaggerated" and held momentarily. There is very little mouthing of *words*. Signs and phrases are often repeated for emphasis: "YOU-GO-FINISH, WHY?...WHY?" ("*Why* did you go?")

One way to "tune into" ASL is to try to catch the

sentence subject. In ASL, the subject, the topic of the sentence, often comes first. Modifiers (such as adjectives) often come AFTER the subject. Signed-English systems follow the syntax of spoken English, and thus place verbs and modifiers before the subject. This makes signed sentences more difficult to "read."

Chapter 15

What is Total Communication?

otal Communication ("TC") seems to have become one of the most misunderstood, misinterpreted, and misapplied terms in contemporary usage.

TC, as a term, was first used by educator Roy Holcomb in 1968. As an alternative to the inflexible oral/aural approach, TC quickly caught on. Although certainly popular in the U.S. and abroad, notably the Scandinavian countries and Australia, TC has proven bit tricky to define. The Conference of Educational Administrators Serving the Deaf (CEASD)[1] defines TC as "a philosophy incorporating the appropriate aural, manual, and oral modes of communication in order to ensure effective communication with and among hearing-impaired persons." It "refers to the right of the deaf individual to have easy access to a wide spectrum of useful forms of communication. However, most people who use the term mean the method of communication used by deaf students that combines both speech and sign (or fingerspelling)."[2]

TC is thus a throwback to an earlier outlook, a broader view which held that the acquisition of speech is not the be-all and end-all of deaf education, just one aspect of it.[3] As a philosophy, TC was something of a breakthrough—a belated recognition that deaf children had the right to access to any form of communication that they felt comfortable with and would benefit from. Obviously, this should include ASL, but in practice, ASL is still extremely rare in the classroom. "Signing" in the classroom almost always means some form of Manually

Coded English (MCE) such as SEE[2] (Signing Exact English).[4]

TC is inaccurately used to mean "simultaneous communication" (a.k.a. "sim-com"), a method of signing while talking. (Sounds easy, but it isn't—it often ends up as a badly tossed salad of spoken English and broken signs.) TC is *also* used to describe oral schools. We recall seeing a newspaper item about an oral school in Israel. A teacher was quoted as saying (more or less), "We believe in total communication. We train the children not to rely on sign language alone." (Meaning, of course, that sign language is discouraged there.) TC has become, it seems, a fashionable euphemism for "oral."

According to the TC philosophy, attention must be paid to the individual needs of each deaf child. This calls for top-quality teaching and flexible programs. A child who has a fair amount of residual hearing may be happiest in an oral/aural program, while one who is profoundly deaf may be happiest in a Signing environment. This is the ideal. The reality, as we all know, is another matter entirely![5]

---

[1] Formerly called The Conference of Executives of American Schools for the Deaf.

[2] "Total Communication," **Gallaudet Encyclopedia of Deaf People and Deafness**, 3:173-175.

[3] How old is the idea of combining modes, anyway? Very old. The earliest oralist teachers employed fingerspelling and some form of sign language to teach speech and writing. This was true even at the famed Braidwood Academy, which held the monopoly on education of the deaf in the English-speaking world (particularly England and Scotland) for 3 generations.

During their first 60 or so years of U.S. schools for the deaf, ASL was freely used both inside and outside of the classroom. (This is the period we refer to as the "Golden Age.") The ascendance of oralism in the late 19th century brought a much more narrow, rigid outlook. All forms of manual communication (including fingerspelling) were banished from the classroom. Signing—any form of signing—was prohibited.

Edward Miner Gallaudet, the founder and first president of Gallaudet University, believed in the "combined approach"—ASL used in the classroom, but with optional classes in oral articulation for those who might benefit from them. Recognizing that the educational tide was turning against Sign, he saw the combined approach as a sensible compromise. In those days, speech training was *optional*. Previous experiments with articulation classes in Signing schools had shown that very few (if any) congenitally deaf children derived any significant benefit from them.

4 There have been numerous attempts to teach English through Manually Coded English (MCE)—invented sign systems which represent English vocabulary and grammatical structure. Perhaps the best-known are SEE¹ (Seeing Essential English), SEE² (Signing Exact English), and Signed English. (Signed English is the simplest and most flexible of these systems.) They were developed in the late 1960s and early '70s for classroom use. Each MCE system has special signs for aspects of English grammar that are not found in ASL—prefixes like *un-*, suffixes like *-ness* and *-ment*, participles (*-ing*), particles like *a, an,* and *the*, verbal past tense (*-ed*), etc. Many root signs are liberally borrowed from ASL, with these invented elements grafted onto them. The effect is odd. These MCE systems have created controversy in the Deaf community. Many Deaf people don't feel that they promote good English skills; they're confusing and unnatural. Signed English certainly has its uses. Communicating with hearing people who don't know ASL is one such use.

5 The label "Total Communication Program" is no guarantee of quality. Parents should check out any TC program before enrolling their child. One English family's experience is instructive. Lorraine Fletcher, seeking a Signing nursery-school environment for her deaf son, Ben, investigated two schools for the deaf. One was oral; the other committed to TC. But she found remarkably little difference between the two schools in what went on in the nursery level. The emphasis was on spoken English. There were no Deaf teachers or assistants. And there were few deaf children. Most were hearing. **(Ben's Story: A Deaf Child's Right to Sign**, pp. 140-143.)

The newest trend in deaf education, the "Bilingual-Bicultural" approach, is a more radical departure from traditional practice; it uses ASL to teach English. It is closer to the original ASL-in-the-classroom mode first used in Hartford in 1817. TC should not be confused with the "Bi-Bi" approach. The two have different aims.

Chapter 16

I heard that ASL is the 3rd most used language in the U.S. If this is true, why don't all universities accept ASL as a foreign language?

We asked Dr. Sherman Wilcox at the Department of Linguistics, University of New Mexico, Albuquerque, NM, an authority on ASL as a second/foreign language. He has some pertinent comments:

 irst, I'm not sure that the figure, "third-most-used language," is correct. But, really, if it is not the third it is pretty high up there and the point is still correct. Why don't most universities accept it? I think because of very deep-seated misunderstandings about what ASL is, also, probably, some not very nice prejudices. My experience is that the belief that ASL can't be a foreign language is based on lack of knowledge of the facts about the language. People have some preconceptions, assumptions about ASL, and then they use good logical thinking to come to conclusions about whether ASL is a foreign language, but because they had faulty preconceptions their conclusions are wrong. So even though people will often say they realize ASL is a language, they don't really fully understand the truth of that statement. They just sort of mouth the words! So, typically, a university professor will say, "Well, it's not a language." Of course, that's not true. Then they will say, "Well, it's not foreign; it's used in this country." But of course, many languages are used only in this country and still are accepted as foreign languages. Here at my university, Navajo is accepted as a foreign language.

It's a very good question and so interesting because it really goes to the heart of people's understanding of what ASL is. It really brings out strong feelings. You know, I can predict now pretty accurately what hearing people will say in reaction to a proposal to accept ASL as a foreign language. First is the "It's not a language" argument, then "Well, it's not foreign." I joke sometimes that "foreign" is in the eye of the beholder. After all, to my American Indian friends here in New Mexico, we Anglo-English speakers are the foreigners. Then people will say, "There is no culture." Well, we can prove them wrong on that one pretty easily. Then they will say, "There is no written literature in ASL." This is a little tougher and I prefer to spend some time going into detail on it. I prefer to first answer: Yes, you are correct. There is no written literature in ASL, but there *could* be. ASL can be written. Writing systems have been designed for ASL but the community of ASL users hasn't accepted them yet, and maybe never will. But in principle, it is possible and really is no different from, again, my pet example, Navajo. Fifty years ago, people could not write Navajo. A man created a writing system. Now some Navajo people can read and write Navajo. Many cannot. Some think it is good; many think it is silly. Just like the Deaf community. And of course many Navajos are bilingual—Navajo and English. Same as Deaf people. So when we talk about literature it is important to recognize that for a bilingual community the literature can be in two languages. Then, after that, I think, is the time to bring up videotape, etc., as ways of sharing ASL literature.

▲ ▲ ▲

According to Dr. Wilcox's fact sheet on ASL as a foreign language (and other sources), some of the colleges and universities which formally accept ASL in fulfillment of foreign or second-language requirements include Bowling Green State University, California State University at Hayward, Centralia College, College of Staten Island, East Central University (Oklahoma), Madonna University, Michigan State University, SUNY Stony Brook, University of Arizona, University of California, University of Minnesota, University of New Mexico, University of Rochester, University of South Florida, University of Washington, and William Rainey Harper College—"the list grows daily! Harvard and Yale are among some of the schools which are [also] investigating [this]."*

Which states officially recognize ASL as a foreign language? At press time, there were 20 such states: Alaska, California, Connecticut, Florida, Illinois, Iowa, Kansas, Louisiana, Maine, Maryland, Massachusetts, Michigan, New York, Ohio, Oklahoma, Pennsylvania, South Dakota, Tennessee, Texas, and Washington.

*Dr. Sherman Wilcox, "American Sign Language as a Foreign Language: Fact Sheet." Albuquerque: Department of Linguistics, University of New Mexico, ca. 1991.

Chapter 17

Why do so many Deaf people have trouble with English?

ecause English is primarily a spoken language. All hearing children of English-speaking parents absorb it unconsciously, starting from the moment they're born. They're surrounded with English; bombarded with it from all sides! They listen; they imitate. Effortlessly, it seems, they begin to put together grammatically correct sentences well before they learn to read. Children who are born deaf (or early-deafened) are excluded from this process because they cannot hear. The lucky ones whose parents are fluent in ASL start school already knowing a language. Those whose parents cannot (and will not) sign are often forced to start school without any real language at all. This can have disastrous effects on their educational development. As Deaf educator Sam Supalla has pointed out, you can't learn a language in the classroom unless you already know a language.

Moreover, ASL is grammatically "at odds" with English. The two couldn't be more different. English is an eclectic Indo-European language, a rich hybrid of Anglo-Saxon syntax, Old French, Old German, a generous measure of Greek/Latin vocabulary, retaining a wealth of grammatical quirks and irregularities. ASL is not a simple string of word-pictures in the air, it's a visual/gestural language—a *very* different approach to communication from a spoken one. For example, ASL has plural forms, but *not* in a recognizably "English" sense. As Harlan Lane points out, "Body shift, sign reduplication, sign trajectory, using more fingers, and using more hands are all devices to indicate various kinds of plurals." ASL does not convey plurals with word endings, nor ongoing activities with participles, nor has it any use for other features that make good English *good English*.

Various forms of manually coded English (SEE[1], SEE[2], etc.) are commonly used in the classroom to teach English. But they have not *really* succeeded in solving the Deaf-literacy problem. They presuppose a working knowledge of English grammar which many deaf children lack. A native ASL user often ends up writing English as though it conformed to the logic that governs ASL. The result: a barely literate pidgin.[1]

A few determined born-deaf persons acquire fluency not only in ASL but also written English. It takes years of agonizing work. It's possible. But rare. Most Deaf people have such a wretched experience with English that by the time they graduate from school with "minimal language skills," they're glad to have done with it. And that's the level of skill they maintain for the rest of their lives. It has nothing to do with intelligence. English is not their first language. ASL is. This is the crux of the ongoing English 50 controversy at Gallaudet University: should the English-proficiency requirements be eased, or should Deaf students be forced to struggle with a language which is not theirs?

Endless difficulty with English has certainly affected the quality of Deaf people's lives—not only their ability to enjoy reading, but their careers, their mobility, their access to information, and their relations with the hearing world.[2] This is *not* a new predicament. It started several generations ago. The blame lies with a society that equates communication with speech, and an educational system that devotes far too much time to oral/aural training while prohibiting ASL in the classroom.

And the Deaf community should share the blame for not having fought harder to prevent this from happening.

Instead of asking only why so many Deaf people can't read and write English, we should also be asking why so many hearing people, especially teachers and parents of deaf children, know nothing about ASL.

1 It *is* possible to teach English through ASL—the "Bilingual-Bicultural" approach. See Chapter 15.

2 Some Deaf adults remain poor readers, but to preserve their dignity ("save face"), try to fake comprehension. Faced with the task of reading and critiquing a piece of writing they don't understand, they'll pretend to understand and appreciate it, reacting with approval, even enthusiasm ("Good!"). Of course, this can get them into trouble. But so deep is their pride, they're willing to risk the embarrassment of getting caught rather than confess their inadequacies beforehand.

Chapter 18

Why don't some Deaf people like to read?

 few reasons:
(1)—ASL is the native language of many Deaf citizens here, and ASL has no written form.

(2)—It was long considered more important for deaf children to acquire good speech articulation than good reading and writing skills. So speech was stressed above literacy. More time was spent on articulation than education. The results? A community with extensive oral training that they have little occasion to use, and a distressingly low level of literacy.

(3)—The attitude of the educational establishment: contempt for/ignorance of ASL, low expectations for deaf students, and a "brutalist" approach to beating the essentials of English grammar into their heads.

The two most common misperceptions about Deaf people and reading are actually two sides of the same coin:

(1) **The Silent Bookworm:** Some hearing people have the misconception that all Deaf people instinctively adore books because the avenue of sound is closed to them. Deprived of music, the radio, conversation, don't they *love* to read? In their frequent isolation, don't books become their only friends?

(2) **The Illiterate Dork:** The other side of the stereotype is equally pernicious: some Deaf people can't read because they're not as intelligent as hearing people, period. They lack mental stimulation; they can't think

abstractly.

The facts: Both of these perceptions are romantic non-sense. Deaf people are social creatures who enjoy a variety of experiences—yes, even going to discos. If books play little or no part in Deaf people's lives, there must be a reason. It is NOT lack of intelligence or some deficiency in the ability to handle abstract concepts. There are a number of Deaf people who are fluent in ASL, yet enjoy reading. If English has been taught to them in a positive way, they can appreciate English literature as much as any native English-speaker. Literacy skills are not a true gauge of intelligence.

Our quarrel is not with the English language as such, but the way it has been (and still is being) taught. No matter how beguiling or potentially enriching the subject, a bad teacher can turn the students permanently against it in no time at all. We all know this. Teachers whose underlying message is that deaf kids *can't* are the prime culprits. Boring, outmoded, and irrelevant material, hateful classroom experiences, and the suppression of the child's native language are not limited to deaf schools, but the consequences are just as destructive. The kids get lost very soon. If they never get beyond "bad, mad, pad, and dad" or drills in sentence diagrams, they won't stick around to appreciate the delights of Jane Austen or Shakespeare. Why bother?

As for the "beauty of the English language," it's been battered forcibly into their heads. Many deaf children have started school without any real language. The common-sense approach would be to give them an immediate grounding in a visual language, then use that language to teach English as a second language. English is *not* a visual language; it's primarily an aural one. But what if ASL was not used or recognized by the teachers? Suppose only a signed form of English—not

ASL—was acceptable? The traditional deaf-ed approach was to drill them, drill them, drill them in English grammar. Could the kids appreciate something they've never understood—much less enjoyed?

What about taking a few minutes to browse through the books in the library? Wouldn't that tempt them? For a bright hearing child, a library is a repository of knowledge, a quiet place to read, to browse, to daydream, a pleasant interlude in a noisy, stressful day. For generations of deaf children, the library was where you got sent as a punishment for misbehaving. Small wonder that many Deaf adults have bad memories (if they remember at all!) of what went on inside their classrooms, and feel absolute indifference to anything that smacks of libraries, literature, poetry—tools of the oppression they were subjected to.

And then there's the ordeal of speech therapy and speech training. Is speech a gift? The birthright of all deaf children? Many deaf children who endured the endless hours of training would have been pleased to decline such a gift. Endless hours spent on auditory training, listening skills, and speech—and their articulation was still poor.

In earlier times, it was not that uncommon for therapists to strike young deaf children. Because they were misbehaving? No, because they mispronounced a word when they repeated it. A word they couldn't even hear.[1]

One Deaf man attributes his distaste for reading and writing English to his classroom experiences:

I hated what went on in my classes. The teachers were hearing. I felt they looked down on us. Always criticizing our writing—'wrong this, wrong that.'

Imagine a class of 30 black kids with a white man teaching them. The kids normally use Black English. The teacher instructs them in correct standard English. Do they bother listening? Even if this white teacher is married to a black woman, it doesn't matter. It doesn't make him black. White teacher, white attitudes. Put a black teacher up there teaching those same kids correct English—that would be different.

Same thing with deaf kids. If we had a Deaf teacher who understood what it means to be Deaf, how a Deaf person thinks, it would have been different. A Deaf teacher would understand our heads. Such a teacher could use ASL to teach English—ask us to describe something or tell a story in Sign, accept our signing, give us positive feedback, then explain the rules, teaching us how to improve our writing. Constant interchange. That'd be good.

Having a black wife doesn't make a white man Black. Learning how to sign doesn't make a hearing person culturally Deaf. (That is, unless they are VERY, VERY convincing—e.g., if their parents were Deaf.) My teachers looked down on the Deaf. Even if they signed, they looked down on us, they had a Hearing attitude. Patience isn't the factor. Attitude is.[2]

We'd like to emphasize that this view, although it represents one Deaf man's opinion, is necessarily simplistic. Not all Deaf teachers make good English teachers! We know of another Deaf man who majored in English at a West Coast university and taught briefly at Gallaudet, who proved to be a notably incompetent English teacher. Sure, he's Deaf—but he just doesn't have the right quality. And vice versa. Quite a few hearing teachers (who had Deaf parents and shared the "Deaf experience") have been outstanding English teachers.

Perhaps attitudes are changing, but the damage has already been done. First deaf children are denied access to their own language in the classroom. They are often under the sway of teachers and administrators who don't know ASL and have contempt for it. English (oral, written, and signed) is used as a tool of oppression. The library is turned into a place of punishment. They are schooled in low expectations. And then they're criticized for doing badly in English and hating to read! Grown, they are penalized by Hearing society for being illiterate.

The literacy skills of Deaf adults generally remain at a third- to fifth-grade level. Small wonder that among many grassroots Deaf, English is relegated to a second-class, crudely utilitarian mode of everyday communication—TTY conversations, occasional notes and letters. Used, but not cherished.

Deaf people do like magazines, particularly those with lots of pictures. **People** and **Us** are very popular; they're heavily illustrated and the stories are brief. Newsmagazines may be scanned for the pictures, but not read. Too inaccessible. Some Deaf people enjoy **National Geographic**, if only to browse through its glorious color photo-essays. Some do read newspapers, for the sports coverage. Many Deaf viewers watch but don't understand TV captioning—it's a barrage of incomprehensible advanced (and occasional phonetically mangled) English whizzing by.

We personally know one Deaf guy who bought a new set of **Encyclopaedia Britannica** that he proudly displayed in his living room—and never read. That's equivalent to hearing people displaying foreign-language classics on their bookshelves, to impress the visitors. This guy also belonged to a sci-fi book club and read the stuff, but didn't really understand what he was reading. And his written English was, well, typical. Most Deaf people are more honest about their distaste for reading and writing English. And you really can't blame them for feeling that way. They've suffered plenty.

[1]On brutal speech therapists: The source for this statement is our own personal experience. In all fairness, it should be noted that modern speech therapists are a better-educated, more sensitive breed than the previous generation. They are trained to treat young deaf children with respect. Anyone caught abusing children would most likely lose her/his job in short order.

[2]A free adaptation of an informal interview in Sign.

Chapter 19

Doesn't closed-captioning help Deaf people improve their English?

here's no denying that closed-captioning is wonderful. However, we need to ask just how much Deaf people are getting from it—certainly a pertinent consideration. Some Deaf people honestly prefer interpreters on TV. (A few programs, notably Christian and Catholic-oriented ones, feature them in fairly unobtrusive oval "inserts" in the lower right-hand corner of the screen.) There are definite advantages to this. Captioning is best appreciated by those with a reasonable degree of fluency in written English—a fluency many Deaf viewers simply do not have. They feel more comfortable with ASL than written English. In rendering audio to written text, captioning functions like a newspaper article being unscrolled—flat words, with no particular emphasis. In contrast, a TV interpreter's signs, facial inflections, and rhythm can convey a much clearer visual sense of what's being said.

There is a basic disagreement within the captioning industry itself: whether to display captions that are a simplified translation of the audio "script," or captions which are a verbatim (word-for-word) transcript. Advocates of verbatim captioning feel that it's unethical and insulting to alter the wording; Deaf and hard-of-hearing viewers deserve to read exactly what's being spoken, no more, no less. Advocates of simplified captioning argue that many Deaf viewers cannot comprehend some of the vocabulary on TV. By simplifying the text, they're making it accessible. The argument isn't likely to be resolved, at least soon. (At this point, verbatim captioning seems to be more widespread.)

Closed-captioning has the potential to increase English skills among Deaf viewers, but there's no hard-and-fast evidence that it's happening yet. From our own experience, we've seen Deaf viewers with typical reading skills watching ABC's captioned *World News Tonight*; when asked about what they've just seen, they say they don't fully understand what's going on. So it's safe to say that at least some of the captioning is simply incomprehensible to many Deaf people. There is, moreover, the troublesome fact that some real-time captioning, about 10%-15% by our estimate, reads as a meaningless phonetic garblemush—"deny airings" for "teenagers," for example. (It happens every night.)

Glasnost, *perestroika*, "rapprochement," "trade embargo," "sanctions," "aggressiveness," "pessimistic," "impasse," "conservative," "liberal," "middle-of-the-road," "recession," "covert operation," "ethnic unrest," "money-laundering scheme," "qualitatively speaking," "clear the decks," "preemptive strike," "dispatched an emissary," "limited endorsement," "stealth candidate," "drug czar," "skullduggery," "miscarriage of justice." Such foreign loan-words, "ordinary" words, phrases, idioms, and occasional slang in common currency on the nightly news, are all outside the normal Deaf usage. To see is not *necessarily* to understand.

Deaf Awareness: 5-Minute Quiz

Chapters 11—19

Answers are on the bottom of the page, upside down.

True or False:

1. Native Signers like to fingerspell large portions of their everyday conversation to stay in practice.

2. Some programs which label themselves "Total Communication" may not even have fluent Signers on the staff, nor offer access to sign language.

3. Edward Miner Gallaudet advocated the "Combined Method"—the use of Signed instruction in the classroom, and training in speech for those who could profit from it.

4. A native American language (like ASL or Navajo) can nonetheless qualify as a "foreign" language.

5. Deaf people hate to read because they have difficulty thinking abstractly.

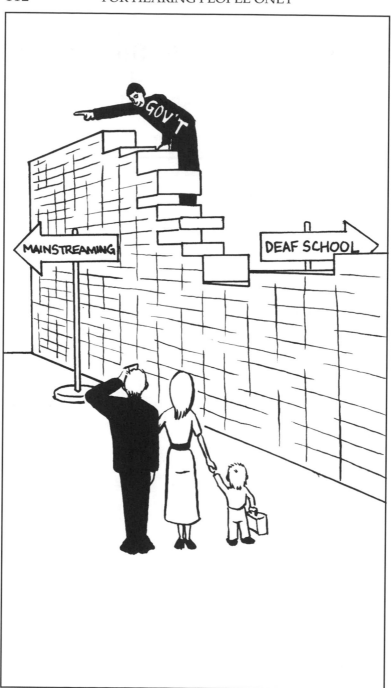

Chapter 20

Why is there a movement to close down residential schools for the deaf in this country?

esidential schools have managed to survive the onslaught of oralism, declining enrollment, and other major challenges, although many are experiencing troubled times. One giant problem is money. Not all residential schools for the deaf are state-run; some operate with very little government funding. Even so, state budgetary cuts are threatening the quality of their programs.

Mainstreaming sounds like a great, inexpensive alternative to costly state-run schools. Save the taxpayers money, right? P.L. 94-142, the controversial "mainstreaming law," has proven a real headache in the way it has been applied. It was not originally intended for deaf children. It was designed to ensure that handicapped/disabled children's individual needs were taken into consideration for the most appropriate placement. Instead, it became an easy excuse to shift deaf children wholesale from residential schools into local day programs or public schools. Dr. Frank Turk, the distinguished Deaf administrator, identifies three major weaknesses in the law: placements are routinely made without adequate input from trained professionals; certification and accreditation standards are lacking; and there is no provision for centralized and early-intervention programs.

Understandably, many parents want their deaf kids to be "normal"—to talk like everybody else and to go to local schools as "normal" children do. As Dr. Peter Seiler argues, there shouldn't be any more stigma attached to attending a state school for the deaf than to a prep school.* But the prospect of sending little Susie or Tom to a state-run institution terrifies some parents. Especially if their fantasy of the state school for the deaf is a Dickensian mill churning out an endless parade of illiterate, unskilled dorks.

Parents *like* to have their kids going to nearby schools and coming home every afternoon. As far as deaf kids are concerned, most mainstream programs haven't been notably successful. True, *some* mainstreamed deaf children thrive. But many feel isolated. (Ask them.) Staffs are not necessarily trained to serve their particular needs. Teachers often cannot communicate with them. Their participation in sports and extra-curricular activities is usually curtailed. Even with an interpreter, they are at an automatic disadvantage.

Closing the state schools and placing all deaf students in local programs is false economy. Conscientious administrators (and not necessarily just the deaf ones!) are dedicated to strengthening residential schools as a viable alternative to mainstreaming. Good residential schools offer advantages no mainstream program can: an abundance of trained professional staff, individual attention, a 24-hour learning/social environment, everyday exposure to ASL, equal participation in *all* activities, and Deaf role models. Any existing communication barriers between the children are swiftly leveled. Many alumni of these schools remain close friends with each other throughout their lives. They see themselves as a community, akin to family—they are all deaf together, sharing the same experiences, challenges, and language. They have generally positive feelings about their education. Many deaf parents of deaf children know that this is the learning environment they want for their own kids.

Choosing the best placement for a deaf child is no easy decision. Parents have to weigh the pros and cons of residential-versus-mainstreaming, for there are pluses and minuses to each. One problem the residential schools have long been struggling with is lower expectations. Many residential schools are simply not as academically challenging as their hearing counterparts. They may have difficulty attracting the best teachers, setting up the most stimulating curricula, and offering the highest-quality programs. Traditionally, graduating deaf students as a whole have scored significantly lower in academic achievement levels than their hearing counterparts, particularly in English skills. The better schools do narrow the gap considerably. We know of no residential-school programs for gifted deaf students.

Granted, schools for the deaf are a very mixed lot. Some have well-deserved reputations for academic excellence. Some just don't have terribly good track records at turning out literate, "quality" graduates. Some have gotten embroiled in sex-abuse or physical-abuse scandals. But the fact is that they fill a vital need, and without the deaf schools, Deaf identity and culture would quickly become extinct. As the 19th-century oralists knew, strike at the deaf schools, and you strike at the very foundation of the Deaf community.

There may be a threat, but there is a backlash at work. The future of the schools depends heavily on the support of the Deaf community. It is important that Deaf constituents organize and make their views known to their legislators. On the other front, the Deaf community needs to *enlist* not only hearing parents of deaf children (who are often our staunchest allies), but *educate* the teachers, the whole deaf-educational establishment itself, and the professionals who make their living ostensibly serving the needs of deaf children—and *this* is the biggest challenge of all.

*"I believe that the proper name for residential schools for the deaf should be the 'state school for the deaf' or any other name similar to this. The school for the deaf has a dormitory only as a convenience to the parents because of the distance for most hearing-impaired children. There should be no stigma attached to attending a state school for the deaf which is no different from attending a private boarding school." **DEAF LIFE**, September 1991. Dr. Seiler is superintendent of the Illinois School for the Deaf, and is deaf himself. He and Dr. Turk were quoted in this cover feature on 12 deaf superintendents/directors of schools for the deaf. There are now some 16 of them in the States—an encouraging trend.

▲ ▲ ▲
"'Hearing parent' is not a dirty word"

*As originally published in the September 1991 issue of **DEAF LIFE**, the concluding sentence read: "On the other front, the Deaf community needs to educate hearing parents of deaf children—and this is the biggest challenge of all." Shortly afterwards, we received a poignant letter from Barb and John Boelter, parents of a deaf child, objecting to this statement. Their view makes an insightful counterpoint to ours. We published it in full in our "A Few More Words" department (August 1992), and are reprinting it here.*

As the hearing parent of a deaf daughter, 18 months old, I must take exception to your response to the question regarding residential schools in "For Hearing People Only" in the September issue. Other parents I have spoken with share my views.

We have known that our daughter was deaf since she was 5 months old. Since that time we have learned more about deafness, deaf education and Deaf Culture than some parents learned in a lifetime. Your comment, ". . . the Deaf Community needs to educate hearing parents of deaf children—and this is the biggest challenge of all" is insulting to parents like us who have recognized from the beginning that our daughter needs the support and guidance of the

Deaf community to grow and find her own identity. We have sought out and listened to the advice of deaf people in connection with every decision we have made.

We are trying to pave new ground in our local schools by pushing for bilingual/bicultural education. Our daughter spends 2 days a week with a deaf family to learn ASL in its natural environment and see successful deaf adult role models. We also participate in as many Deaf Community activities as possible.

I know that hearing parents years ago cannot be blamed for believing "experts" who told them not to sign with their kids. I think I understand why older deaf people feel such strong ties to their residential schools. But on the other hand, parents today who do recognize the social, educational and emotional needs of their deaf children should not be penalized for what parents didn't do in the past. "Hearing parent" is not a dirty word and deaf people as a group should be more sensitive to this type of stereotyping.

I do not want a residential school to be the only option for a quality education for my child. With a stimulating home environment and participation in the Deaf Community, she will be able to achieve her potential and learn about Deaf Culture while in the family setting. Any child should learn life's really important lessons at home, i.e., values, self-worth and unconditional love. A school should provide only part of a child's educational and social needs.

Perhaps if deaf parents were told over and over again that they were not able to provide an appropriate environment and identity for their hearing children, they would understand our frustration.

Give hearing parents a chance. Work with us, not against us, to get the best possible education in all settings. With the help of our deaf friends, we will raise happy, educated and proud deaf children who will be a credit to both cultures.

Respectfully submitted,

Barb and John Boelter
Eagan, Minnesota

[P.S.] I realize that this may be longer than most of your letters but please publish it as I feel it represents a viewpoint that may not be known to many deaf adults. They may feel their Culture is at stake, but my child is at stake and until someone faces that situation, you cannot understand.

Thank you.

Chapter 21

What's the best clearinghouse for information about deafness?

he best place to start is your local public or school library. Depending on size and location, they're likely to have at least a few basic books on deafness and sign language, and possibly some periodicals of interest. Ask the reference librarian to help get you started in the right direction. (See the bibliographic listings at the end of this book.) **The Encyclopedia of Deafness and Hearing Disorders** (Facts on File, 1992) has 13 useful appendices—listings of community programs, agencies, organizations, performance groups, supervised housing, summer camps—even "Where to Learn Communication Skills." Perhaps your library has a copy of the 3-volume **Gallaudet Encyclopedia of Deaf People and Deafness**. If not, ask if they can borrow it through interlibrary loan.

The best overall resource center, and a good starting point if you have a fairly clear idea of which direction you want to go, is the **National Information Center on Deafness** at Gallaudet University (NICD). Its address is 800 Florida Avenue N.E., Washington, D.C. 20002. ☎ 202-651-5052 (Voice/TTY). Did you know that Gallaudet has a bookstore at the same address, and a mail-order catalogue featuring a wide variety of books and publications on deafness? You can order these (not just Gallaudet University Press publications either) through the catalogue.

Also try FOLDA (Friends of Libraries for Deaf Action): P.O. Box 50045, Washington, D.C. 20091-9998, USA. ☎

202- 727-1186 (Voice); ☎ 202-727-2255 (TTY).

The Deaf Counseling, Advocacy and Referral Agency (DCARA) is a well-known organization. Its motto is "Of, by, and for the deaf." Headquarters are at 125 Parrott Street, San Leandro, CA 94577. ☎ (510) 895-2430 (Voice); ☎(510) 895-2432 (TTY).

The **National Association of the Deaf** (NAD), whose headquarters are at 814 Thayer Avenue, Silver Spring, MD 20910, also features a mail-order catalogue. ☎ 301-587-1788 (TTY). Another possibility is the **GLAD Bookstore**, 615 S. Westmoreland Avenue, Los Angeles, CA 90005. ☎ 213-383-2220 (TTY). Besides Gallaudet University Press, several publishers, notably T.J. Publishers, DawnSignPress, and Sign Media, specialize in Deaf Culture- and ASL-related material. ASL is particularly suited to the medium of videotape. DawnSignPress, for example, produces ASL videotapes as well as books; Sign Enhancers specializes in ASL videotapes.

Addresses and TTY and fax listings for many local and national Deaf organizations, institutions, agencies, clubs, businesses, as well as many Deaf people, all handily arranged by state and by category, can be found in TDI's **International Telephone Directory for Text Telephone Users**. It's also known as the "TDI Directory" or the "blue book." TDI (Telecommunications for the Deaf, Inc.) is located at the same address as NAD. ☎ 301-589-3786 (Voice); ☎ 301-589-3006 (TTY). Ask your library for a reference copy of the directory.

For questions pertaining to law and deafness, try the **National Center for Law and the Deaf**, also at Gallaudet University (7th and Florida, N.E., Washington, D.C. 20002).

For medical aspects of deafness, try **The Encyclopedia of Deafness and Hearing Disorders** (Facts on File), or contact the Deafness Research Foundation.

Schools and colleges for the deaf are good resources, too. For example, try NTID (National Technical Institute for the Deaf, P.O. Box 9887, Rochester, NY, 14623-0887).

And keep in mind that Gallaudet, NTID, CSUN (California State University at Northridge), NAD, TDI, the Alexander Graham Bell Association for the Deaf, SHHH (Self Help for Hard of Hearing People, Inc.), the Association of Late-Deafened Adults (ALDA), and GLAD (Greater Los Angeles Council on Deafness) all publish magazines and other useful material, such as reprints and pamphlets.

Happy hunting!

Chapter 22

"My wife teaches children with learning problems. Would there be any information to help her better recognize children with hearing problems or anything related?"

Through my [ASL] courses, my wife has been able to help hearing-impaired children (at least to recognize their problems) and a child who's hearing but his parents are deaf. The little boy speaks okay, but sometimes he reverts to an English version of the ASL sentence structure. Teachers were beginning to think something was wrong. He was merely translating into spoken language the language he was raised with. My wife is helping him learn the written English now.* She teaches children with learning problems.

Would there be any information to help her better recognize children with hearing problems or anything related?

R. M.
Wheaton, Maryland

here's certainly no shortage of information—the problem is deciding where to start excavating. Some books which may prove useful are listed in the bibliography in the back of this book. New ones are coming out all the time.

The libraries of NTID/RIT, CSUN, and Gallaudet are prime resources. RIT's Wallace Memorial Library, for example, has free bibliographic lists on several relevant topics. E.g., "Recent Acquisitions in DEAFNESS" is periodically updated and includes listings of new reference and circulating books, all with Library of Congress call numbers. Several dozen theses on microfiche are also listed.

As for organizations and agencies: Do a bit of riffling around in the current **TDI Directory** (official title: **International Telephone Directory for Text Telephone Users**). Start with national organizations such as the National Society for Deaf Children, AGBAD, and TRIPOD. Also try GLAD (California). Then zero in on the local, county, and state agencies.

Since this question was originally asked by a resident of Wheaton, Maryland, we referred him and his wife to the Maryland section of the directory. We noted that Maryland, together with Washington D.C., has the nation's heaviest concentration of Deaf organizations and agencies, so there are plenty of listings! Washington has several, too. . .

For example, we suggested Maryland's Office for the Coordination of Services to the Handicapped, and Montgomery County Department of Family Resources—Services to Handicapped Individuals, and encouraged these readers to contact the state school for the deaf—in this case, Maryland School for the Deaf, which might be able to give some useful leads. Ditto the state education agency: e.g., Maryland State Department of Education/ Infants and Toddlers Program.

The National Information Center for Children and Youth with Handicaps (P. O. Box 1492, Washington, D.C. 20013), Beginnings for Parents of Hearing Impaired Children (1316 Broad Street, Durham, NC 27705), and Infant Hearing Resource (3930 S.W. Macadam Ave., Portland, OR 97201-9847) can all provide further information.

Then there's computer networking . . .

And don't forget that trusty resource, the National Information Center on Deafness at Gallaudet University. (NICD provided some of the above leads.) In fact, any readers with similar questions might want to ask there **first**.

A few of the many available works on deaf children, early intervention, and education:

Frank Bowe, **Approaching Equality: Education of the Deaf**, 1991

Katharine G. Butler, **Early Intervention: Infants, Toddlers, and Families**, 1989

Paul C. Higgins, **The Challenge of Educating Together: Deaf and Hearing Youth: Making Mainstreaming Work**, 1990

David M. Luterman and Mark Ross, **When Your Child is Deaf**, 1991

Eugene Mindel and McCay Vernon, **They Grow in Silence** (rev. ed.), 1987

Donald Moores, **Educating the Deaf: Psychology, Principles, and Practices**, 1982

Paul Ogden and Suzanne Lipsett, **The Silent Garden** (rev. ed.), 1991

Mark Ross, ed., **Hearing-Impaired Children in the Mainstream**, 1990

H. Schlesinger and K. Meadow, **Sound and Sign: Childhood Deafness and Mental Health**, 1972

Sue Schwartz, Ph.D., ed., **Choices in Deafness: A Parents Guide**, 1987

Alec Webster, **Children With Hearing Difficulties**, 1989

Robert E. Johnson, Scott K. Liddell, and Carol J. Erting, **Unlocking the Curriculum: Principles for Achieving Access in Deaf Education**, 1989

*For more details on the problems faced by hearing children of Deaf parents, see Chapter 31.

Chapter 23

I've been working with a deaf man for 20 years. He's an excellent lip-reader. Recently I met his friend, who uses sign language. I tried to communicate with him and couldn't. I was shocked. Can't all Deaf people read lips?

ne of the most common "Hearing" misconceptions is that all deaf people have this magic ability to 'read lips.' All too often, the first question a hearing person asks a new deaf acquaintance is, "Can you read my lips?" (Note: This is the *one* question *all* deaf people can undoubtedly speechread!) Even if the answer is "yes," the hearing person will often exaggerate his or her mouth movements and talk abnormally slowly, which of course makes communication that much more difficult. If the answer is "no," the deaf person may be perceived as a poor sport and/or a nitwit, and whatever potential there was for communication will be totally nullified. ("Huh? How can she say no? She answered my question correctly, didn't she? Is she playing games?")

Lipreading involves a high proportion of guesswork and "instant mental replay." Only some 30% of all spoken sounds are visible on the lips. Many sounds, like "b," "p," and "m," are virtually impossible to distinguish by watching the mouth. And what about homonyms (homophones)—"blue" and "blew?" They look *and* sound identical! Moreover, everyone makes sounds a bit differently; everybody's voice and articulation are different. A stranger, whose speech patterns are unfamiliar to the lipreader, presents a more formidable challenge than members of the household or close friends. All this means that even a skilled lipreader must rely to some extent on guesswork to understand what's being said, using the context to fill in the inevitable gaps.

Anyway, 'lip-reading' is a misnomer. A more accurate term is *speechreading*. Speechreaders don't just look at the mouth; they read the entire face: the eyes, the way the eyebrows tilt or the brows knot when certain words are emphasized. They note changes in expression, shoulder shrugs, posture, gestures. They also note any props the speaker is carrying; their surroundings. Picking up these *associational cues* is an art in itself. It requires a high degree of attention. It can be exhausting.

Everybody (hearing as well as deaf) makes use of some degree of speechreading at times. For deaf people, it's a survival skill. Even so, some consider speechreading skill an inborn ability, like dancing. Many deaf people never become very proficient at it. If all else fails, hearing people should forget the "rubberlipping" and try the old standby, pencil and paper.

▲▲▲

Speechreading Protocol:
a few words of advice

Nothing creates so much anxiety in Deaf-Hearing relations, it seems, as the fateful first encounter. A few suggestions to make it a bit easier for all those involved:

1. Facial Topography: Many deaf people who are skilled speechreaders have difficulty "reading" men who have full or unkempt beards and/or thick, sweeping mustaches. Men and women who don't remove sunglasses or doff hats that overshadow their faces also create difficulty for deaf readers. People who nervously shield their mouths with their hands while talking or who take frequent furtive glances to the side, breaking eye contact, drive us crazy. It's best to remain relaxed, focused, and clear as possible.

2. Popping the Question: If you run into a deaf person (and we're assuming that you don't know sign language or fingerspelling, which is the case with the majority of hearing folks), ask politely, in as natural a way as possible, "Can you read my lips?" or "Can you speechread me?" Don't over-enunciate (exaggerate) your question. You don't *have* to point to your lips (but most hearing people do this instinctively); if you do, do it discreetly—don't ham it up, repeatedly jabbing at the air in front of your mouth. You're not auditioning for a third-rate sit-com; you're trying to communicate.

3. What Comes Next: If the deaf reader shakes her/his head or says "No," be friendly. Don't shrug, throw up your hands in dismay, or mumble, "Sorry." And whatever you do, *don't* walk away. Try to establish some common ground. Get a pen and paper. Use a restaurant napkin. Scratch letters on your vertically-upended palm. (Don't bother "writing" letters in the air, however—this *never* works well.) If you want to badly enough, you and your deaf reader will think of *something*. Human beings are a pretty ingenious species. Two persons who have a language barrier and *really* want to communicate will usually find a way.

Chapter 24

"A deaf woman in my office does not speak. However, we do hear actual understandable words from her once in a while. Does this mean that at some time, someone has worked with her in speech? And is it wrong to want her to verbalize?"

I have recently taken a new job with a congenitally deaf woman in the office. As a manager, I felt it necessary to at least try to learn enough to communicate with this woman; enough Sign Language to be fully understood, and, as important, to learn about the deaf and their culture. Needless to say, it has been, so far (several months) a real eye-opener and extremely interesting. I find it hard to believe that this culture and language is so prevalent around us, but, as a hearing person, I knew absolutely nothing about it.

Anyway, I have taken here at work a very basic course in Sign Language. It really didn't get into ASL as such, mostly vocabulary to be put together into Signed English. The woman at my office can understand what little I know. I am presently enrolled at Gallaudet in their beginning ASL course.

The woman in my office does not speak. However, we do hear actual understandable words from her once in a while. Does this mean that at some time, someone has worked with her in speech? And is it wrong to want her to verbalize? I recently read a biography of Gallaudet and understood there are two schools of thought on this subject, but since this woman does work and live in a hearing English-speaking society, is it wrong to want her to be able to speak? Of course, I'm not trying to get her to do this or anything, just wondering.

R. M.
Wheaton, Maryland

t's not *wrong*—it's human nature. Most parents of children newly diagnosed as deaf are terrified at the prospect that little Susie or Tom will never be able to speak. Traditionally, oral schools have emphasized speech training above literacy skills, although the graduates of oral schools don't necessarily end up with better articulation than those from signing/Total Communication schools. Oralists maintain that career opportunities are better for speaking-deaf than for non-speaking (Signing) deaf—an understandable but questionable conviction.

But if speech is the key to success, is non-speech the automatic gateway to second-class citizenship?

Virtually all deaf adults have had a heavy dose of speech and auditory training. It's an inescapable fact of life for deaf schoolchildren, whether the school be residential, state, private, or public. Oral training is part of the "Total Communication" curriculum. As Ken Levinson, former president of the Alexander Graham Bell Association for the Deaf, has pointed out, the quality of this training varies wildly. Many speech-therapy programs have been haphazardly (or downright badly) administered. There are skillful speech therapists—*and* a lot of brutal, ineffectual, plain bad ones—just ask around.

And, obviously, not all deaf children benefit from speech training. Good articulation is notoriously difficult both to achieve and maintain, especially for those born deaf or early-deafened. How well can you modulate your voice if you can't hear yourself speaking? If you have *never* heard yourself speaking? You can never really be sure how you sound—the only cues are the expressions on the faces of your listeners. Or comments such as, "Sorry, I can't understand you" (the polite version), or "Gee, what planet are you from?" (the rude version). A scary thought? Many deaf people have endured plenty of humiliation and pain from the reactions of others to their "strange" voices. They *know* that their voices sound harsh and unpleasant; they're embarrassed about using them.

Some of our most distinguished Deaf leaders, past and present, have never uttered intelligible words. Others (a relative few) are highly skilled speechreaders with good oral articulation. When dealing with hearing non-signers, some Deaf people who prefer not to vocalize, nonetheless try to accompany their Pidgin signing with speech. It's a matter of personal preference, what Levinson calls "comfort level."

As for your wanting your Deaf co-worker to verbalize, that really has to be her decision. If she feels comfortable with it, she will. You can, of course, ask her how she feels about talking with her voice, and what kind of experiences she's had with speech therapy and auditory training during her school years. But speech should never be forced on, or demanded of, deaf people.

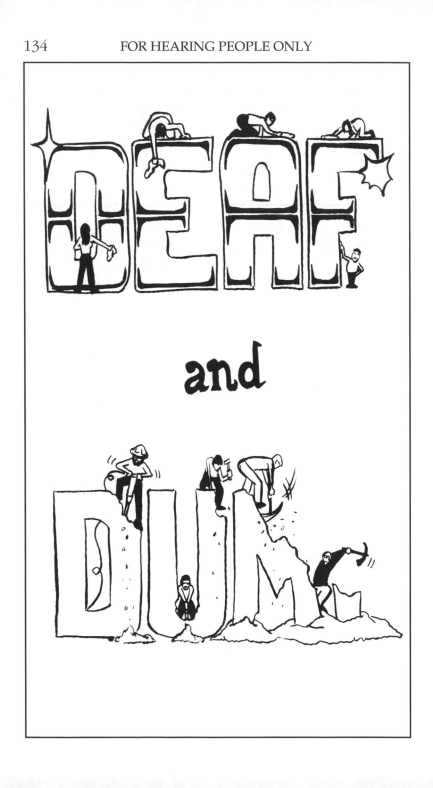

Chapter 25

Is it OK to use the term "deaf-mute" in reference to a deaf person who can't talk?

o, it's no longer an acceptable term. "Mute" refers to someone who *cannot* talk, that is, produce intelligible speech, or someone who has malfunctioning or missing vocal cords. "Mutism" is a medical or psychological condition— the *inability* or *refusal* to produce sounds. Virtually all deaf persons are physically *and* psychologically normal in this area. They have vocal cords and voices, just as the vast majority of hearing people do. This also applies to deaf people who prefer to communicate exclusively in sign language. Their vocal apparatus is perfectly normal. But, being deaf, they cannot hear themselves talk, and thus, cannot easily modulate their voices. Consider: If you were born deaf or became deaf as an infant and have never heard yourself talk, it's extremely difficult to talk clearly, with normal intonation. So signing is the natural mode of communication for many deaf people; speaking can never be. A few deaf people have good clear articulation—better than some hearing people—but most don't. It's a matter of personal preference, deciding what we feel most comfortable with.

Why isn't "deaf and dumb" an acceptable term?

Think about the last time you used the word "dumb." You used it to describe something stupid, clumsy, or foolish, right? A century ago, this term was in common use. Nobody thought twice about its propriety. It's outmoded now, and insultingly inaccurate. We're aware that this term is still used in England to describe someone who is deaf, but that doesn't say much for the discernment of those who persist in using it.

As for the correct term, why not simply say "deaf?"

A note on "politically correct" terms

Originally, the terms "deaf-mute" and "deaf-and-dumb" were not considered pejorative; they simply referred to a severely or profoundly deaf person who didn't speak. "Semi-mute" referred to a moderately deaf person or one who had become deaf after learning how to speak, both of whom could profit from articulation training.

Nobody thought twice about the political correctness of such terminology. The American School for the Deaf was first called "The Connecticut Asylum, at Hartford, for the Education and Instruction of Deaf and Dumb Persons," although, it should be noted, some of the Deaf people involved disliked having "Asylum" in the title. The original name of Gallaudet University was

"Columbian Institution for the Deaf, Dumb, and Blind," then, after it was chartered, "National Deaf-Mute College." (It was renamed "Gallaudet College" in 1894.) The first publication in the "Little Paper Family" (1849) was **The Deaf Mute**. At its 1880 founding, the National Association of the Deaf called itself "National Convention of Deaf-Mutes." No disrespect intended. These terms simply reflected the prevailing 19th-century belief that deafness caused muteness.

Interestingly, it was the oralists who began trying to abolish the term "mute." They made grandiose claims that all deaf children could be taught how to speak. But the Deaf community (who knew better) refused to believe it. They did NOT want to speak, and did NOT want to be identified as speaking deaf. Because the oralists tried to suppress sign language in favor of speech, Deaf leaders preferred to continue calling themselves "deaf-mutes," as it made the oralists uncomfortable. Using the term "deaf-mute" thus became a symbolic act of defiance to the oralists' explicit goal of "making the deaf speak." It was wielded as a cultural badge of pride. As the great Deaf leader George Veditz remarked, "If oral magicians who yank educational rabbits out of silk hats and pearls of speech out of the mouths of those who have never heard, choke over it, why, bless 'em!"

Nonetheless, the terms "deaf-and-dumb" and "deaf-mute" gradually faded from acceptable usage. Sensibilities have changed since Veditz made his whimsical comment. All deaf children now get a stiff dose of speech training (we have the oralists to thank for that), so there is little point in splitting the deaf population artificially into speaking and nonspeaking categories. "Deaf-and-dumb" and "deaf-mute" are now politically incorrect, period.

We dislike these terms because they now convey a

negative attitude. "Deaf and dumb" does not connote pride or wholeness. It conjures a pitiful, pathetic, dull-witted image, with a hint of subnormal intelligence. "Deaf-mute" suggests that a deaf person is doomed to a life of silence, without speech, without hope. We've run into these terms repeatedly, and we find them annoying, inaccurate, and insulting.

How widespread are the terms "deaf-and-dumb" and "deaf-mute"? They seem to be more common in England and Canada than here, although that's not saying very much. We've seen several examples of headlines from the British press that made us cringe, but then, we've seen American headlines that were just as bad. In England, "deaf and dumb" is used to describe even deaf people who can speak clearly. The British Deaf Association has been waging a public-education campaign against this term, and kindly sent us a copy of a pamphlet (aimed at media sub-editors) titled "Deaf People Are Not Dumb."

Some U.S. newspaper and magazine reporters still use "deaf-mute." Possibly they think it adds "color" to the story. "Deaf-mute woman slain" makes the deaf victim sound more victim-like than "Deaf woman slain." "Deaf-mute held in slaying" sounds more lurid and criminal-like than "Deaf man held in slaying."

We have found the term "deaf-mute" in contemporary books (e.g., **A Day in the Life of America**). This is bothersome, because a book's influence is more permanent and pervasive than that of a newspaper. Books are kept. They have influence. Staying power. Once they're published, they stick around. They go onto library shelves. They get borrowed and re-borrowed, read and reread by schoolchildren and adults. And you can't easily fire off a letter to the author that gets published in next Monday's morning edition.

We have also seen these terms on television, not from the anchors or reporters, but from hearing people being interviewed. Actual examples: "He's a deaf-mute." "My neighbor's a mute." "She's deaf and mute and went to the deaf-and-dumb school." A number of hearing people who really should know better are caught using phrases like these. If you're going to be quoted by the press or a TV reporter, please, think twice!

(We'd like to note that **DEAF LIFE** has an occasional feature, "Oh, No! Not Again!", which "showcases" examples of these offensive terms as used in contemporary media. Readers send in examples, and we run across a number of them ourselves.)

So what *are* the correct terms? Understandably, some hearing people find the simple, blunt, four-letter word "deaf" a bit hard to swallow. "Deaf" can mean not only "unable to hear," but "heedless" or "unwilling to listen." Common expressions such as "deaf to their pleas," "their appeal fell on deaf ears," "turned a deaf ear," and "the silence was deafening," have a decidedly negative connotation. To some people, "deaf" still connotes something shameful. Recent euphemisms include "hearing-impaired," "hearing-handicapped," "hearing-disabled," "auditorily handicapped," and "non-hearing." Most deaf people dislike these terms, as they promote a negative image of deaf people as broken ears or malfunctioning machinery. "Deaf" refers to the medical fact of hearing loss, but can also designate pride and cultural affiliation (i.e., "**D**eaf"). Fussy terms like "auditorily-handicapped" don't.

Some members of our community honestly prefer "hearing-impaired" to the more archaic "hard-of-hearing"—and vice versa. "Hearing-impaired" may be useful as a way of designating all those with various degrees of deafness, including mild, moderate, severe, and profound hearing loss. But those who insist on using this term should best employ it in combination, i.e., "deaf/hearing-impaired/hard-of-hearing." That way, nobody gets left out. The majority of deaf people prefer the simple term "deaf."

We'd like to note that the International Federation of the Hard of Hearing, the World Federation of the Deaf, NAD, and the Pennsylvania Society for the Advancement of the Deaf, have all agreed that the term "hearing-impaired" is no longer acceptable, and that "deaf/hard-of-hearing" should be used in all future references.

▲ ▲ ▲

"Silent" Overkill

Another bothersome word is the cliché "silent." We are aware that there are Silent Clubs, "Silent" athletic teams, and "Silent" publications. "Silent" is a quaint way of indicating that we don't communicate in speech, i.e., that we're deaf. However, some Deaf people find it a bit tiresome, as when the Deaf reality is described as "a silent world." Some of us feel that it simply doesn't apply. True, a gathering of Deaf people may be quieter in terms of vocal noise, but Deaf people are NOT soundless creatures.

Deaf people sometimes accompany their Signed conversation or reactions (e.g., to television) with a variety of grunts, clicks, snorts, whoops, or chuckles. We laugh and cry; we utter sounds to express incredulity or surprise, just as hearing people do. Since we can't hear ourselves, we often have no idea of just how loud we *are*. In a Deaf-culture context (e.g., a Deaf hangout, or an

NTID/RIT dorm lobby), this is not a problem. When we're "in public," that is, among hearing people, this can sometimes get us into trouble.

Deaf people sitting at tables use the table as a signing base, thumping it as part of their Signed conversation, to express a spontaneous reaction, or to get someone's attention. The sign for "right/correct" is one "pointing" handshape (active hand) struck down onto another "pointing" handshape (passive hand). But Deaf people eating and talking together will often dispense with the passive hand and simply strike the sign onto the table. What hearing people hear is a sharp thwack.

To get someone's attention, we stomp on the floor. That can be noisy. What is a normal and acceptable aspect of Deaf culture may be unthinkably rude or gross (i.e., noisy) in Hearing culture. If you're a jittery hearing person living in an apartment just below a bunch of Deaf people, we don't have to educate you about noise. (You have our sympathy.)

"Silent" suggests sensory deprivation, mutism, and isolation, none of which accurately describes the Deaf experience. (When we think of a "silent world," we envision a scuba diver's paradise, complete with coral reefs and exotic varieties of fish.)

If you think of the Deaf world as a silent one, how do you account for the fact that Deaf people like noisy discos, percussion music, loud jukeboxes, and stomp-dancing? We enjoy fireworks just as much as hearing people do. We love the explosions of color, the booming and the crackling.

As applied to the Deaf experience, "silent" *can* be apt, poetic, even amusing. But we think it's misused and overused. "Silence" is like a hot spice—it should be used sparingly. Too much sears the palate, numbs the senses, and spoils the feast.

▲ ▲ ▲

What do others call us?
And what do we call ourselves?

What's in a name? That which we call a rose
By any other word would smell as sweet...
—William Shakespeare, *Romeo and Juliet*

"Sticks and stones may break my bones, but names can never hurt me," goes the old children's rhyme. Many a mother has taught that rhyme to a daughter or son who came home crying after being taunted. Parents have tried hard to convince their children that names aren't important, that they're harmless and can't *really* hurt anyone, and that to respond with tears and fury is to overreact. But life is not that simple. There's no denying that names *are* important, and labels—names applied to a group—can have a profound effect on the members of that group. Labels can build self-esteem. Or they can be used as weapons to degrade and insult. A label influences what we think of ourselves. It creates expectations that are fulfilled.[1] To name something is to have power over it.

As deaf people, we have a vital interest in the labels applied to us by the hearing majority. Labels help us understand the mindsets of those who do the labeling; we can recognize the image others have of us, true or false, and identify stereotypical thinking. We can measure what progress we've made, and gauge how far we have yet to go.

Progress comes slowly. All of us have different opinions—some of us prefer the term "hearing-impaired" to "deaf" or "hard-of-hearing." Some deaf people still insist on using the term "deaf and mute." We need to examine these labels and see why they're used, and by whom, and what image we *really* want to promote. We need to understand them, monitor them, and confront them. When we find these terms still being used by those who should know better, we need to remind the users. We have a right to express our opinions forcefully, to object to the way we're labeled, and to insist on change. And we have the right to choose what we wish to be called.

DEAF AND DUMB/DUMMY
Real-life examples:
*"Look at the **dummies**, talking with their hands!"*—woman in a restaurant, early 1980s

*"Admirers of the **deaf and dumb** actress Elizabeth Quinn will warm to her biography, written in association with Michael Owens, called **Listen to Me.**"*—**Inside London** (a free cultural-events magazine for tourists), August/September 1985

*"By using signs like those used by **deaf-and-dumb** people, scientists have been able to teach several gorillas to express feelings and ideas."*—Michael Fitzpatrick, **A Closer Look at Apes** (New York: Gloucester Press), 1987

*"Ex-**Dynasty** star Emma Samms has dumped another man—this time breaking the heart of a handsome **deaf-and-dumb** actor to whom she had publicly confessed in sign language: 'I love you.'"*—**The Globe** (a supermarket tabloid), October 3, 1989

*"You'd have to be **deaf, dumb and blind** not to want to grow up to be a dynamic, exciting person."*—Frances Cohen,

quoted by Roxanne Roberts in a feature on a gossip columnist, **Washington Post**, July 28, 1990

*"You've proven that love can be not only blind but **deaf and dumb** as well."*—Ann Landers, in her December 5, 1990 column

Dictionary definition:
deaf-and-dumb, *adj. Often Offensive.* deaf-mute (def. 1). [1150-1200; ME *def and doumb*]—**Random House Dictionary of the English Language,** 2nd Edition, Unabridged (1987)[2]

Quotes:
Terminology has a long and sordid history in the world of deaf people. "Deaf and dumb" was the status quo *for many years. People who use it still (yes, some still do) may claim that they only mean "dumb" to indicate that deaf people can't talk, but the word carries with it the definite implication that deaf people are stupid.*—Richard Nowell[3]

I asked my father the next day, "Why do you let them call you Dummy?"

He shrugged, his nostrils still full of cotton from the [upholstery] shop. "I tell them my name is Ben. I tell everyone my name is Ben, but they call me Dummy. It is easier for them. They remember me."

I was enraged. "You are not a dummy. You are my father and a smart man. Tell them over and over that your name is Benjamin."

He smiled wanly, tired with the long day's work. "It is all right. I know I am not dummy, that is enough."—Ruth Sidransky[4]

Our view:

The great-granddaddy of all negative labels. Surprisingly, this was originally a reasonably neutral term.[5] It was based on an ancient misconception that deafness caused the inability to speak—if you were deaf, there was also something amiss with your capacity for speech (and, it followed, if you couldn't speak, you couldn't reason).

Although the vast majority of hearing people now know that deaf people have perfectly normal vocal apparatus, the usage still persists. We've found recent examples in England, Canada, and the States. The British Deaf Association, for example, has been conducting an ongoing campaign to educate the media and public (and to convince them once and for all to stop using the term), and publishes a pamphlet, "DEAF PEOPLE ARE NOT DUMB: A BDA Guide for Sub Editors on the correct terminology associated with deafness," which provides a concise explanation of why the term "dumb" is offensive, inaccurate, and just plain wrong.[6] In the States, the battle is fought on a newspaper-by-newspaper basis by individuals who write personal letters to editors to try and set matters straight. It's slow going. Despite all the urgings, British newspapers (especially the more lurid ones) seem quite unconcerned about the propriety of the term. And American newspapers will quote interviewees who use these terms, without comment. So "deaf-and-dumb" manages to stay in usage.

The vulgar form of this term, "dummy," is a crude insult. An old nickname for deaf people—athletes, co-workers, neighbors—it's now used by hearing people to mean "stupid." Ernest Tidyman deliberately used it for the title of his book about Donald Lang, the languageless deaf man accused of murdering two prostitutes. He took the most shocking and offensive term he could—

the same term used by other hearing people to describe Lang—to make readers uncomfortable, to make them think about the ways Lang had been labeled all his life.[7] Even so, some readers and TV-viewers have complained about the title, fearing that it promoted the use of an insulting term as though it were acceptable.

People who don't consider themselves prejudiced will utter the most extraordinary things at unguarded moments. In the first example quoted above (told us by a friend), two hearing women sat down at a table in a restaurant and ordered. At the next table sat three friends—two Deaf women and a sign-language interpreter (who was, of course, hearing). They were having an animated conversation in ASL. One of the two hearing women stared at them, nudged her companion and said out loud, "Look at the dummies, talking with their hands!" They snickered. The interpreter overheard this and relayed the information to her friends. They decided on a plan of action. They sat quietly for a few more minutes, then stood up together, turned towards the two women, made identical "Who, me?" gestures (exaggerated shrugs, palms-up), and said aloud, in unison: *"WHAT DUMMIES???"* The two women turned scarlet. They were *so* embarrassed that they got up and charged out of the restaurant right then and there—they didn't even wait for their lunch to arrive. We hope that they learned from it.

DEAF-MUTE
Real-life examples:
"When police arrived, the couple's 5-year-old **deaf-mute** *daughter was mopping up her mother's blood."*—From a story in the Gary, Indiana **Post-Tribune**, March 6, 1990, "Battered wife used the system, was still murdered by

husband," AP byline

3 deaf-mutes murdered in Clifton; baby spared—headline in the **North Jersey Herald & News**, March 26, 1990

*"In December, authorities in Taipei uncovered a gambling ring composed entirely of scores of **deaf-mutes** operating via fax machines."*—Chuck Shepherd, "News of the Weird," **City Paper** (Washington, D.C.), July 1990

*"My father knew a **deaf-mute**. His name was Putt and he was homeless. He lived in a rowboat. Putt had been gassed in World War II and was a strange and mixed-up guy."*— Congressman Joseph P. Kennedy II, interview in the **Boston Globe**, August 9, 1990

Dictionary definitions:
deaf-mute, *adj*. **1.** unable to hear and speak.—*n*. **2.** a person who is unable to hear and speak, esp. one in whom inability to speak is due to congenital or early deafness. [1830-40; trans. of F *sourd-muet*]—**Random House Dictionary** , 1987

deaf-mute also deaf mute. *Offensive.*—*n*. A person who can neither hear nor speak.—*adj*. Unable to speak or hear.—**American Heritage Dictionary of the English Language**, Third Edition, 1992

Quotes:
A person who is deaf cannot hear; a person who is mute cannot make any sounds. Rarely do these two conditions appear in the same person. Most deaf people have fully functional vocal apparatus. They may not speak intelligibly but this has to do with the type of deafness, age of onset, and the type and amount of speech training received in the course

of an individual's education. Speech proficiency has nothing to do with a person's intelligence or linguistic capabilities. Most deaf people who do not speak well are fluent in American Sign Language and literate in written English. To hearing people the term "deaf-mute" is loaded with negative connotations. The Deaf community doesn't need someone of your stature and influence perpetuating the use of this outmoded label.

(. . .) Your description of Putt made deaf people appear childish, helpless and dependent. Sure, Putt was only one deaf person but stories like this form the basis of people's stereotypes.—Kim Schive, Arlington, Massachusetts, letter to Congressman Kennedy[8]

The more recent term, "deaf-mute," may not be quite as bad [as "deaf-and-dumb"], but it is still pretty terrible. Besides being inaccurate, since deafness and an inability to produce voice are not connected, it also leads the general public into many misconceptions. And some people shorten it to just "mute," seemingly losing the whole point about the characteristic of the individual. (I recently heard someone say, "I've got two cousins who are 'mutes'.")—Richard Nowell[9]

Our view:

A hundred years ago, "deaf-mute" was an acceptable term. (Gallaudet University was formerly called "National Deaf-Mute College," and nobody seems to have objected.) At one time, Deaf people were proud to call themselves "deaf-mutes." Oralists disliked the term "deaf-mute;" their goal was to assimilate all deaf people into Hearing society by making them learn how to speak. When the oral method began gaining popularity among hearing teachers, administrators, and wealthy do-gooders, Deaf people resented the grandiose claims that *all* deaf people could be made to speak, and clung to the old term (which the oralists wanted to abolish), to emphasize their political stance: 'We are deaf, and we refuse to be forced to speak.' "Deaf-mute" was thus a term of pride. How times change! The term gradually faded from "acceptable" usage, ironically enough, as the oralist movement gained power over the education of deaf children. By the 1920s, all deaf schools in the States had made the switch (or been forced to switch) to the oral method, so—supposedly—all deaf children *could* be made to speak. No more "deaf-mutes." Gradually, the term became obsolete—but it has never completely disappeared.

Today, even in schools where sign language is used freely, virtually all deaf children get a stiff dose of speech therapy and auditory training, so the old distinction between speaking and non-speaking deaf has become moot. We all know (don't we?) that it is extremely difficult, if not impossible, to modulate your voice if you can't hear it. If deaf people prefer not to speak, it's not because they *can't* speak but because, being deaf, they can't properly modulate their voices. Whether or not a deaf person speaks intelligibly is largely a matter of choice—an individual decision based on comfortable they feel about vocalizing.

What was once a "reasonable" term has become degrading. "Deaf-mute" no longer means "proud non-speaking Deaf signer." It now carries a negative connotation, suggesting the pathetic, subhuman, mentally backward, helpless. That's why the vast majority of deaf people dislike it.

It's a fact of life that labels help to sell newspapers, especially tabloids.[10] "DEAF-MUTE WOMAN FOUND SLAIN" is more lurid, more shocking, than "BRONX WOMAN FOUND SLAIN." It makes her more of a victim. The general reader reacts more strongly to

"DEAF-MUTE MAN JAILED" than to "CHICAGO MAN JAILED." A "deaf-mute man" seems more threatening, more sinister, than "Chicago man." It's a cheap trick, but an old one. We hasten to add that not all ists are irresponsible and insensitive. According to the standards of the Associated Press (AP), "deaf-mute" is NOT acceptable, and thousands of newspapers in the States comply with these standards. Media coverage, when done in a sensitive, thoughtful way, has done much to increase "Deaf awareness" throughout the world, and we applaud it.

Nonetheless, a distressing number of newspapers, radio talk-show hosts, police departments, etc., still think "deaf-mute" is an acceptable term. Or they don't think at all.

DEAF AND MUTE
Real-life examples:
"My wife and I are both **deaf and mute** *(please, not 'deaf and dumb') and we use sign language to communicate with each other."*—From a letter by "J.J.P. in Baltimore," in "Dear Abby," early December 1990

"Rachelle has had quite a hard life because of her disability. She's **deaf and mute** *and went to the* **deaf-and-dumb** *school. Rachelle's extremely hard-of-hearing, so anyone who gives her an ounce of love, she'll pay back in tenfolds."*—Leo Tessier of Canada, talking about his daughter, on **Unsolved Mysteries**, February 19, 1992

Our view:
As the first example shows, even intelligent, sensitive people (deaf as well as hearing) fall into the trap of thinking that "deaf and mute" is an acceptable term.

(**TIME** Magazine still uses it.[11]) Ironically, "J J P in Baltimore" was sharing a "old but true" story about a sophisticated deaf gentleman who meets an ignorant hearing man on a train and gets the better of him in a positive and good-humored way, and obviously wanted to show readers of this extraordinarily popular column that deaf people were intelligent and sophisticated!

As for the second example, it's sad to see ignorance so nakedly displayed, on prime-time TV, yet.

MUTE
Real-life example:
*"My neighbor's a **mute** and there's a man in her house."*—Odessa Ray of Chattanooga, Tennessee, re-enacting the 911 call she made on behalf of her deaf neighbor, Annette Armour, in **Rescue 911**, March 27, 1990[12]

Dictionary definition:
mute—*n. Offensive.* One who is incapable of speech.—**American Heritage Dictionary**, 1992 (one of several meanings)

Our view:
A term used by uneducated people. On **Rescue 911** a few years ago, we saw a re-enactment of how a deaf couple with no TTY coped with a housebreaker at night. The mother (fluent in ASL) grabbed her hearing son (also fluent in ASL) and ran next door. The boy told the neighbor what was wrong. This neighbor immediately phoned 911 and said by way of explanation, "My neighbor's a mute." Question: why couldn't she have said, "My neighbor's deaf," and saved a bit of time? Exactly how does "mute" equal "deaf"? "Mute" means refusing or unable to speak. This suggests that some

hearing people still see deaf people solely in terms of their supposed inability to utter articulate sounds.

We now leave traditional terms and move onto modern ones. "Deaf-and-dumb," "deaf-mute," "deaf and mute," "mute"—these terms are part of our past, symbolizing the way society viewed us.[13] We're not advocating that they be expunged from dictionaries, nor do we advocate bowdlerization of historic accounts. All we ask is that these terms be recognized as obsolete. They are inaccurate and, therefore, offensive. We've moved beyond them, and we need to move beyond the others as well.[14]

HEARING-IMPAIRED
Real-life examples:
*"Teaching sign language to **hearing-impaired** children is 'akin to child abuse,' according to Gerry McGrath, an educator of the **hearing-impaired**."*—**The Advertiser** (an Australian newspaper), April 17, 1990

*"Janice Wuertz, a sign-language interpreter for the **hearing impaired**, started daily finding herself at age 32 fighting off 'sleep attacks' during the day."*—John G. Hubbell, "New Help for Troubled Sleepers," **Reader's Digest**, September 1992

*"There is a clear need in the United States for improved methods and models for early identification of **hearing impairments** in infants and young children. Approximately 1 of every 1,000 infants is born deaf. Many more children develop some degree of **hearing impairment** by the age of 3. Reduced hearing acuity during infancy and early childhood interferes with the development of speech and language skills.*

Moreover, delayed identification and intervention may impede the **hearing-impaired** *child's ability to adapt to life in a hearing world or prepare for life in the* **hearing-impaired** *community.*"—William H. Hall, Director of Communications, Office of Medical Applications of Research, Public Health Service, February 5, 1993[15]

Dictionary definitions:
hearing-impaired, *adj.* **1.** having reduced or deficient hearing ability; hard-of-hearing: *special programs for hearing-impaired persons.*—*n.* **2.** (*used with a plural v.*) hearing-impaired persons collectively (usually prec. by *the*).— **Random House Dictionary,** 1987

hearing-impaired *adj.* **1.** Having a diminished or defective sense of hearing, but not deaf; hard of hearing. **2.** Completely incapable of hearing; deaf.—**hearing-impaired** *n.* (*used with a pl. verb*). Persons who are deficient in hearing or are deaf: *the speech was interpreted in sign language for the hearing-impaired.*—**American Heritage Dictionary,** 1992

Quote:
At recent meetings of the International Federation of the Hard of Hearing, World Federation of the Deaf, National Association of the Deaf, and Pennsylvania Society for the Advancement of the Deaf, it was agreed the term "**hearing-impaired**" *was no longer an acceptable term, instead future references would be to deaf/hard of hearing.*—Lillian Hoshauer, Manager, Deaf-Hearing Communication Centre, Inc., Springfield, Pennsylvania[16]

Our view:
A modern euphemism[17] for "deaf." Now quite common, but much resented. Note that the dictionary defi-

nitions are contradictory (reflecting confusion in usage). As the first three definitions suggest, it's not really equivalent to "deaf"—it means "hard-of-hearing," more or less. Deaf and hard-of-hearing people are two distinct groups with different aims, although they do share a common need for accessible communication (e.g., captioning, telephone access). "Deaf" and "hard-of-hearing" are not synonymous, but those who use "hearing-impaired" seem to think so.

The phrases "sign-language interpreter for the hearing-impaired" and "interpreted in sign language for the hearing-impaired" are fairly common usage. It doesn't make sense to us. "Hearing-impaired" people do not use sign-language interpreters. Deaf people do. (And since sign language is the basis of Deaf culture, you might as well capitalize that "D.")

As noted above, the World Federation of the Deaf and other organizations agreed in 1991 that the term "hearing-impaired" was no longer acceptable usage, and that references should be to "deaf/hard-of-hearing." Unfortunately, a lot of people haven't yet gotten the message.

At any rate, "hearing-impaired," *not* "deaf/hard-of-hearing," seems to be the preferred term in the medical field. "Deaf" has a decidedly negative connotation[18] among the rehabilitationists. They may not give a reason, but they clearly prefer to avoid using it.

"Hearing-impaired" defines deaf people solely in terms of broken or defective ears. The same hearing people who prefer "hearing-impaired" to "deaf" tend to be professionals in the audiological-rehabilitation field who take a narrow medical view of deaf people: that deafness is a deficiency that needs to remedied with auditory devices, therapy, and implants. Hearing loss is something to be "aided" or "corrected." Deaf ears are malfunctioning mechanisms to be fixed. Deaf persons are consumers of expensive devices to make them more "normal."

Can you imagine a "National Theatre of the Hearing-Impaired"? We can't. "Hearing-impaired" ignores all positive aspects of deafness: the Deaf community, language, and culture. Rehabilitationists don't want to recognize these, anyway.

We dislike "hearing-impaired" (and its "aurally-handicapped" variants) because it categorizes deaf people as broken machines. This label makes us seem less independent, less capable, less human. The emphasis should be on the person, not the impairment; on what we *are*, not what we lack.

Not all habitual users of the term are in the medical field, of course. We've gotten many press releases from "mainstream" companies that have done commendable things like setting up TTY lines, training personnel in the fine points of deaf-hearing communication, and hiring and promoting deaf people. However, a number of these companies (or at least their press-release-copy-writers) persist in using the term "hearing-impaired," carefully avoiding the word "deaf." When **DEAF LIFE** publishes these press releases, we generally edit out the term, unless there's a good reason for keeping it. Three examples of unedited press releases:

*According to UL Vice President Jim Beyris: "With the new UL Standard and the first UL Listing of smoke detectors designed specifically for them, the **hearing-impaired** community can now increase their safety through the use of these* detectors." (fall 1992)

Hearing-impaired consumers will be able to reach Royal Caribbean to request brochures and have questions answered. Hearing-impaired consumers wishing to book a Royal Car-

*ibbean cruise will be asked to contact the local travel agent of
their choice.*

*"We recognize the need for booking and information sys-
tems which are readily accessible to the **hearing-impaired,**"
said Rod McLeod, Royal Caribbean's executive vice president
of sales, marketing and passenger services."* (mid-Novem-
ber 1992)

*Said John Story, Executive Vice President for British Airways
USA: "This enhancement enables British Airways to reach a
growing part of the traveling population. As a customer-
responsive and caring airline, it recognizes the need to provide
the necessary communications link to all **hearing-impaired**
individuals, who now have an easier time arranging their
travels in order to experience British Airways' high-quality
products and customer service."* (winter 1992)[19]

What would these corporate executives think if they
realized that the term they use so freely is offensive to
the majority of the very people whose patronage they're
trying to attract?

Some folks seem to think "hearing-impaired" is a
more polite term than "deaf." But there is nothing
unpleasant or undignified about the term "deaf," so no
polite substitute is needed.

True, "hearing-impaired" doesn't pack the offensive
wallop of "deaf-and-dumb" or "deaf-mute." It *is* negative and annoying. We don't run into the old negative
terms all that often, but we run across "hearing-impaired" every day. Trying to set matters straight on an
offender-by-offender basis can be exhausting—an endless task. However, we, as Deaf people, possess a sense
of humor. We can turn the tables on those who label us.
An ad for Flying Words Project, an ASL-poetry perfor-

mance, read "Voice-interpreted for the sign-language-impaired."

HEARING-HANDICAPPED
Real-life examples:
*"Making technology accessible to the **hearing handicapped"***—HEAR NOW's old motto, circa 1989. It now reads: "Making technology accessible to the hearing impaired."

*"Gallaudet students have **hearing handicapping** conditions."*—From a United Methodist News Service press release, September 4, 1991

Quote:
*On February 1, 1993 we changed our name from the Association for the **Hearing Handicapped** to* CONNECT SOCIETY. *We also changed our slogan to* Deafness, Education, Advocacy, Families... *which forms the acronym,* DEAF.

Why the change? Because our stakeholders didn't feel that our old name said enough about what we do and what we stand for.—announcement from CONNECT SOCIETY, a community-based agency in Edmonton, Alberta, Canada

Our view:
A cute way of saying "deaf" while avoiding the word "deaf." Excuse the pun, but this sounds like doublespeak.[20]
Again, we don't like being categorized as a group solely on the basis of our hearing deficit. We are not *that* handicapped—most deaf people don't have a physical disability that interferes with their mobility. It's society that *makes* us handicapped by keeping so many opportunities inaccessible and refusing to learn how to com-

municate with us. The majority of our deaf readers don't even consider themselves handicapped.[21] We don't think in terms of deficit but wholeness.

AUDIOLOGICALLY HANDICAPPED
Real-life example:
*"A coalition of business and community leaders, chaired by Nevada First Lady Sandy Miller, herself a teacher of the **aurally handi-capped**, will spearhead the fundraising drive."*—From a November 1989 press release about a caption-decoder campaign in Nevada[22]

Our view:

More doublespeak. This label includes variations like "aurally handicapped," "auditorily handicapped," and "auditorially handicapped"—fancy medical-sounding replacements for "deaf." Again, Deaf people resent this emphasis on broken auditory equipment.

One of the government-funded National Institutes of Health is called "National Institute on Deafness and Other Communication Disorders." This is profoundly ironic in light of the fact that Deaf people, who use a sophisticated visual-spatial language, have contributed greatly to our understanding of communication.

HEARING-DISABLED
Example:
*The **hearing-disabled** community will ben-efit from the ADA.*—(We've seen something like this around somewhere)

Our view:

Modernization of "hearing-handicapped." We still come across occasional references to "hearing-disabled individuals" or "the hearing-disabled community." Since "disabled" has become a popular replacement word for "handicapped," euphemisms for "deaf" take a parallel course, logically enough. How far can you take it? Current replacement terms for "handicapped" are "physically challenged" and "differently abled." We haven't seen "audiologically challenged" or "differently-hearing-abled" yet, but at the rate things have been going, it's just a matter of time, isn't it?

Richard Nowell proposes the term, "persons with hearing loss," to include both deaf and hard-of-hearing. He says, "Alternatives like 'hearing-challenged' seem very stilted to me."

HEARING-DEFECTIVE
Examples:
*Improved technology brings new hope to **hearing-defective** individuals.*—(See comment on previous example)

*"Children of **defectives** often feel guilt."*—Psychiatrist at a large oral deaf school, to Lou Ann Walker, daughter of Deaf parents, circa 1976[23]

Our view:

Disabled people were known as "defectives" in the old Soviet Union. We don't know what terms they use now, but we hope they're less chilling than this.

Likewise, we hope that the psychiatric/psychological profession in the United States has cleaned up *its* act.

NON-HEARING

Real-life example:

*"The National Theatre of the Deaf combines the spoken word with sign language to create a visual language theatre that is enjoyed by both hearing and **non-hearing** audiences."*—

Southern Bell pamphlet

Quote:

*In referring to Deaf people as "**non-hearing**," Southern Bell reduced Deaf to a sterile, sub-average population. Better that they should say "**hearing-impaired**"—even that cringe-inducing term is less debasing than "non-hearing." Perhaps they should use the terms "**Deaf**" and "**non-Deaf**." Wouldn't that be something?*—Stacey Bradford, Flagler College, St. Augustine, Florida, in a letter to Southern Bell[24]

Our view:

A colloquial replacement term for "deaf." It tries to avoid the negative connotations of "hearing-handicapped" and "hearing-impaired." Unfortunately, it's still a negative term—it describes deaf people in terms of what they're not—rather like saying "nonwhites" to describe Blacks.

CAN'T HEAR

Real-life example:

*"Goldie **can't hear**!"*—written by a Kansas City orthodontist's nurse on a deaf woman's medical-history form, 1984

Our view:

Not so bad, but not so good, either. Nowhere near as offensive as "hearing-impaired" or "hearing-disabled," this term still carries a slight whiff of the negative. The word "can't" has long been employed as a deadly weapon against the dreams of deaf children. ("You can't do that, you're deaf.") We prefer to accentuate the positive. Also, the label "can't hear" is misleading, as it implies that it's simply a matter of loudness, that shouting will remedy the problem. It doesn't.

DEAF

Real-life example:
*"Beginning in January 1993, all of the classic episodes of the long-running CBS series M*A*S*H are accessible to **deaf and hard-of-hearing** television viewers."*—The Caption Center, from a press release, February 16, 1993

Dictionary definitions:
deaf, *adj.* **1.** partially or wholly lacking or deprived of the sense of hearing; unable to hear, **2.** refusing to listen, heed, or be persuaded; unreasonable or unyielding: *deaf to all advice.*—*n.* **3.** *(used with a plural v.)* deaf persons collectively (usually prec. by *the*). [bef. 900; ME *deef*, OE *de[e]af*; c. MLG *d[o]of* ; D *doof*, OHG *toub*]—**Random House Dictionary**, 1987

deaf *adj.* **1.** Partially or completely lacking in the sense of hearing. **2. Deaf.** Of or relating to the Deaf or their culture. **3.** Unwilling or refusing to listen; heedless: *was deaf to our objections.*—**deaf** *n. (used with a pl. verb).* **1.** Deaf people considered as a group. **2. Deaf.** The community of deaf people who use American Sign Language as a primary means of communication. [Middle English *def*, *deaf*, from Old English *de[e]af*]. USAGE NOTE: Some critics have lately introduced a distinction between the lowercase noun *deaf*, which is used to refer simply to people with extreme hearing disorders, and the capitalized noun *Deaf*, which refers to the culture and community that has grown up around the use of American Sign Language as a primary means of communication.— **American Heritage Dictionary**, 1992

Quotes:
"Deaf people can do anything . . . except hear."—Dr. I King Jordan, first deaf president of Gallaudet University, 1988

For the sake of clarification in identifying people, why don't we use one word—DEAF—for those of us who are deaf, hard-of-hearing, and deafened, with no measurement of our hearing loss? Let's look at ourselves as one People with our sub-cultures....Let's use the word—DEAF—which is a simple word that everyone understands universally. (Please don't use **'Hearing-Impaired'** *on us as it is a classically negative and medical term.)*

If you, the readers, don't like the simple word—DEAF— why don't you make a survey and ask deaf people to come up with a better word? I tried a new word—"Seeing"—once before, but it did not work out at the time....My point was that we could get together and pool our thoughts to come up with a better word. **WE** *can change words... It is time to develop a better and more simple word to define us: deaf, hard-of-hearing, and deafened people.*—Julianna Fjeld, response to Stacey Bradford[25]

There are three words I'd love to see eradicated from the English language: "handicapped," "disabled," and **"hear-ing-impaired."** *Those three words make it look like there's something wrong with me and I am not normal. I resent that very much! Who gives the hearing people the right to decide who's normal or who's not? I like the term* **'deaf'** *because it is non-judgmental.*—A reader[26]

Our view:

Our readers have told us that they overwhelmingly prefer "deaf" because it's a simple, non-judgmental term. In a "Faxview" opinion poll, 90% of our respondents said they preferred the term "Deaf," 1% "Hearing-Impaired," and 8% identified themselves as "Hard-of-Hearing."[27]

Terms like "hearing-impaired" and "non-hearing," in their narrowness, exclude the possibility of a language and culture; "deaf" is inclusive. So why doesn't everybody use the term? If we have a solution, why is there still a problem?

Some hearing people are squeamish about using the word "deaf." It makes them shudder inwardly. (Could it be because it sounds like "death?" One of us once got a letter from an uneducated hearing friend saying, "I thought you were death...") Or they avoid the term because they feel it's not dignified. After all, one of its meanings is decidedly negative: "refusing to listen." Or they feel it's crude—*deaf* is a 4-letter word. They prefer fancy-sounding terms like "hearing-impaired," which sound more polite, softer—deodorizing an "unpleasant" reality.

Do we need to have this reality deodorized, however? What's wrong with saying "deaf" to mean "deaf"? *Why* is "deaf" considered a dirty word? *Why* do so many companies advertise services and TTY numbers for "the hearing-impaired" when they could save 12 characters of precious ad space by saying "deaf"?

Traditionally, deaf people have been regarded with fear and hostility. There was something strange, even scary, about deaf people. They were considered cursed, devoid of a soul, creatures to be pitied. Even today, there is something taboo about deafness in American culture. A common response to a fearful topic is denial. This carries over into our language and, of course, advertising, which tells consumers what they want to hear (excuse the pun). Who wants to admit that they're going deaf? So they say, "I have difficulty hearing," or "I have a slight hearing loss," or "I have a moderate hearing impairment." Nobody out there in mainstream-advertising-land, it seems, is willing to use the 4-letter word.[28] An ongoing advertisement in **Reader's Digest** for a popular in-the-ear hearing aid reads, "I'm *not* deaf!" Righto.

What Deaf people have been doing, in a variety of ways and mediums, is to stand up boldly and tell the world, "We're deaf, and it's all right to be deaf. We have a history, a language that is the source of our culture, a heritage, an ethnic identity. We have a folklore and a sense of humor. We are human and whole. Many of us communicate differently from hearing people, but we are just as normal as hearing people consider themselves to be."

Deaf can be a positive identity. Deaf is another way of being human. And "Deaf" is what *we* prefer to be called.

WHAT NEXT?

Quote:

"The [British] media views deaf people as defective, pathetic, people who need help. Obviously, the press thinks deaf people are second-class citizens....

"We all know the media is important because of awareness, publicity, but it goes far beyond that; it involves a question of public attitude. Attitude is looked on as one of the biggest barriers to true integration, and also helps influence the individual's personality. If the media portray deaf people in a negative, labeling way, that is passed on to the hearing society, who will then pass it on to deaf individuals.

"If we don't change people's attitudes towards deaf people,

*we will never be equal, never. Before we do that, we've got to
sort it out, make it clear about who we are, how we define
ourselves. Then we can move together with courage, strength,
and conviction, and take on the media."*—Doug Alker,
Director of Community Services for the Royal National
Institute for the Deaf, London, England, "Misconceptions of Deaf Culture in Media and the Arts," presentation, The DEAF WAY Conference, July 1989.[29]

DEAF LIFE now uses "deaf" and "hard-of-hearing."
(Actually, that's been our practice for some time.) We
leave quotations containing terms like "hearing-impaired" when we feel they're absolutely necessary; otherwise, we edit them out. You can help spread the word
by telling your friends and colleagues that "deaf" and
"hard-of-hearing" are the preferred terms.

Whenever you come across an offensive label in a
newspaper, magazine, TV or radio talk-show interview,
advertisement, or everyday conversation, confront the
users. Write a letter to the reporter, editor, newspaper,
magazine, station, company, or ad agency explaining
why the term shouldn't be used, and what the proper
terms are. Use your own words, and be polite. Your local
public library can help you track down the addresses
and the names of the "top brass." (In "Oh, No! Not
Again!" and "Letters to the Editor," we've published
several letters of complaint which can serve as models.)
Remember, labels *can* become obsolete. Dictionaries
and editorial style sheets *can* be updated. People's attitudes *can* change. We *can* do something about negative
labels by taking a positive approach.

NOTES
[1] We now know that labels ("slow-track," "backwards," "gifted")
can directly affect a child's sense of self-worth and performance.

We recall one experiment in which a group of "below-average" schoolchildren were re-labeled "academically gifted." As if by magic, their performances improved.

2 The **American Heritage Dictionary** contains no listing for "deaf-and-dumb."

3 "I'm Training You to Teach Students Whose Ears Don't Work Right," eighth installment of "The Way I Hear It," **DEAF LIFE**, December 1991.

4 **In Silence: Growing Up Hearing in a Deaf World** (New York: St. Martin's Press, 1990), pp. 192-193. This incident took place in 1940.

5 See, for example, Mark Twain's **Huckleberry Finn** (1884). There are two "genuine" deaf characters in the book—Jim's hapless daughter Lizabeth and the English gentleman William Wilks—and one character who fakes deafness (the "duke").

6 "Letters to the Editor," **DEAF LIFE**, August 1992.

7 Ernest Tidyman, **Dummy** (New York: Bantam, 1975), "Author's note." A TV-movie adaptation, also titled *Dummy*, premiered in 1979, and got excellent reviews.

8 "Oh, No! Not Again!" **DEAF LIFE Plus,** January 1991. Congressman Kennedy is the son of Robert F. Kennedy, assassinated in 1968.

9 "I'm Training You to Teach Students Whose Ears Don't Work Right."

10 **tabloids**: smaller-size newspapers with emphasis on brief, sensationalistic stories focusing on crime, violence, and sexual scandal, instead of "serious" news. E.g., the **New York Post** and the **Daily News**, as opposed to **The New York Times**.

11 **TIME's** cover story, "Death by Gun," (July 17, 1989) included a brief account of Patrick Kappus and his daughter Emma, of Brunswick, Georgia, both shot to death on May 1, 1989. Mr. Kappus and his wife were described thus: "a deaf-mute...she is also a deaf-mute." One of our readers wrote a letter of protest to **TIME** and got a response. **TIME** told her that the briefs had been taken directly from police reports. So the police evidently described the victims as "deaf-mutes," and **TIME's** writer copied it. **TIME** apologized to the reader. (See "Letters to the Editor," **DEAF LIFE**, March 1990.) However, **TIME** was soon at it again. An article on Max Ernst by the famed art critic-historian Robert Hughes in the April 22, 1991 issue contains a reference to "a school for deaf and mute children."

12 "Captionwatch," **DEAF LIFE Plus**, May 1990.

13 "Deaf-and-dumb" and "deaf-mute" don't have visual coun-

terparts; there is no corresponding phrase, "blind-and-dense." This reflects the fact that blind people have traditionally commanded more respect from society. There *are* parallel euphemisms: "visually-impaired," "visually handicapped," "non-sighted," "can't see," etc. Most blind people prefer the term "blind."

[14] A few deaf people dislike the old term "stone-deaf," used to refer to someone who's profoundly deaf. See Mary J. Thornley's objection to "stone-deaf" in "Oh, No! Not Again!", **DEAF LIFE Plus**, December 1991. Most deaf people don't seem to consider this offensive, though.

The adjective "silent" is sometimes used inaccurately to describe the Deaf community and communication. "Silent" isn't necessarily a negative word, but if it's used as a euphemism for "deaf," it *can* be.

[15] News Briefs, **DEAF LIFE Plus**, April 1993.

[16] "Letters," **DEAF LIFE**, November 1991.

[17] A **euphemism** is a "good" or "polite" word used as a substitute for a "bad" one—to soften or mask an unpleasant truth, or make something sound better: "passed away" instead of "died," "pre-owned" for "secondhand" or "used," "sanitation engineer" for "garbage collector." Contemporary English language is full of euphemisms.

[18] **connotation**: the underlying meaning or implication of a word beyond its literal sense. Consider some of the different words for "fat": "overweight," "adipose," "heavy," "large," "gross," "corpulent," "portly," "bulging," "fleshy," "full-figured," "matronly," "lard-bucket," "fatso," "out of shape," "porcine," "plump," "obese," "beefy," "chubby," "buxom," *"embonpoint,"* *"zaftig"*—all have different connotations. Some are considered rude, others polite. Some are used as euphemisms. Some are crude slang terms, some medical, others humorous or even affectionate.

[19] These examples were published (all in edited form) in our December 1992 and January 1993 News Briefs (UL—12/92, p. 20; Royal Caribbean—12/92, p. 15; British Airways—1/93, p. 22).

[20] **doublespeak**: language that is deliberately vague, misleading, or inflated. Examples: "air support" instead of "bombing;" "precipitation activity" for "rain;" "covert operation" for "burglary;" "revenue enhancement" for "tax increase."

[21] See "Faxview: Readers' Responses," in **DEAF LIFE**, February 1993: "Do you consider yourself handicapped?" 87% of our respondents said no; 13% yes.

[22] News Briefs, **DEAF LIFE Plus**, January 1990.

23 Lou Ann Walker, **A Loss for Words** (New York, Harper & Row, 1986), pp. 150-151.

24 "Oh, No! Not Again!" **DEAF LIFE Plus**, August 1991. Q.v. Julianna Fjeld's response, "Letters," **DEAF LIFE**, December 1991: "We at the National Theatre of the Deaf are very respectful and appreciative of Southern Bell for sponsoring our performances. The unfortunate choice of words in their promotion in no way lessens the fantastic work they do on the artistic and cultural levels. Southern Bell has long been recognized for its involvement with and support of the deaf community." The term "non-hearing" was probably the work of a copywriter working from NTD/Southern Bell press kits who thought "non-hearing" sounded more "genteel" than "deaf."

Deaf people aren't the only ones with an "image" problem. Consider the current question: what should we call older people as a group? What's a dignified but honest term that *everybody* can accept? *Elderly, aged, old-timers, retirees, over-60's, Golden Agers, senior citizens?* Many people hate being called "senior citizens." Not all older people are retired. And so forth.

25 "Letters," **DEAF LIFE**, December 1991.

26 "Faxview: Readers' Responses," **DEAF LIFE**, February 1993.

27 "Faxview: Readers' Responses," **DEAF LIFE**, December 1991.

28 Well, not exactly. Companies like The Caption Center and Merrill Lynch, which specialize in or have departments catering to Deaf consumers, correctly use the word "deaf" in their ads. But "deaf" is notably absent from other companies' ads aimed at the mainstream market.

29 **DEAF LIFE**, October 1989, p. 29.

Authors' note: This chapter addendum is an adaptation of **DEAF LIFE's** May 1993 cover story.

Deaf Awareness: 5-Minute Quiz

Chapters 20—25

Answers are on the bottom of the page, upside down.

True or False:

1. Residential schools for the deaf are the best placement for *all* deaf and hard-of-hearing children.

2. All deaf people develop a remarkable talent for lipreading.

3. At one time, the terms "deaf-and-dumb" and "deaf-mute" were not insulting. Most people believed that deafness caused muteness, so these terms simply reflected prevailing belief. Even deaf people used them.

4. The adjective "silent" is especially descriptive of the Deaf reality, since deaf people communicate quietly and never make noise.

5. Some people dislike using the word "deaf," even when they're describing culturally-Deaf people, because they feel it's not polite.

Chapter 26

What do you call a deaf person who doesn't speak?

ou call her or him a Deaf person, that's what. Back in the not-so-good old days, hearing folks felt the need to make a distinction between deaf persons who "could talk like a normal person" and those who didn't. Those who didn't speak were branded "deaf-mutes" or "deaf-and-dumb."[1] Is it a question of the *inability* to speak? Hardly. We have yet to meet a deaf person who doesn't have the full complement of vocal equipment. And ALL deaf children, no matter what kind of school they attend, are subjected to an intensive regimen of speech therapy and auditory training. (Some, of course, refuse to continue. But many do because their parents insist on it.) This means that, technically, virtually all deaf children *can* speak.

It is estimated, however, that a congenitally, profoundly deaf child has, at most, a 5% chance of developing intelligible speech. We have to be realistic. Because they cannot hear themselves talk, profoundly deaf people cannot control the pitch, inflection, or loudness of their voices. Some have had humiliating experiences when they tried to "talk normally" in public and were greeted by screwed-up, disdainful faces that said, "Ugh, you sound like a freak!" From our own observations, the quality of a deaf person's intonation has little, if anything, to do with the kind of education they've received—oral or Sign-based. We've met alumni of the Clarke School, the best-known oral school in the country, who have become full-time Signers and whose voices are just as unintelligible as any other deaf voice.

Paradoxically, deaf children whose first language is Sign tend to develop better speech than those who are given intensive early oral training without exposure to Sign. Why? Having a solid foundation in a visual language (i.e., ASL) makes it easier for the child to pick up another language—i.e., spoken English. Such children are more confident in their speech than those without the early exposure to sign. All along, the oralists have been warning parents that if their deaf children learn to sign first, they'll never develop coherent speech! Hogwash.

Developing "normal" intonation is, however, a long, arduous task for a deaf child. The value of these hundreds (thousands?) of hours of auditory/speech training is questionable in some cases, especially when the adult chooses not to speak. Deaf-rights advocates are not against speech training as such; they feel that the time could be much more fruitfully employed in developing good English skills—reading and writing, that is.

A person who is hard-of-hearing (mildly to moderately deaf) or late-deafened will generally have much clearer speech than one who is born deaf or early-deafened. It is unfair to compare the speech skills of those who are born deaf or early-deafened with those who had the advantage of having been able to hear their own voices for years!

To speak or not to speak? It's strictly a matter of personal preference and comfort. Every deaf person is an individual. If s/he feels comfortable using his/her voice, we say fine. But a good number of deaf people do not, and we insist that their feelings be respected. Hence the complaints about Marlee Matlin's 1988 Oscars "speech." Matlin has always used her voice, enjoys it, feels confident enough to take speaking roles, and stays in training. But how typical is she? Most Deaf people don't have the luxury of a Hollywood articulation coach and feel oppressed when their bosses/friends/parents ask them, "If Marlee can talk so nicely, why can't *you*?"

Speech is a survival skill—useful in some situations, but optional. Many Deaf people lead full, productive, happy lives without it—and they deal with the Hearing world every day. Bernard Bragg (who, by the way, does *not* use his voice) has a touching anecdote in his autobiography, **Lessons in Laughter**, about entering Fanwood[2] knowing all the sounds except "k"—the one sound his Deaf mother had never learned to make and couldn't teach him. Having struggled to master this sound in his articulation class, he insisted on teaching his mother how to make it. He drilled her relentlessly until she could say "k." Now, he writes, she could go into a luncheonette and order a cup of coffee.

[1] Some British and Canadian people (including newspapers) still persist in using the obnoxious term "deaf-and-dumb" to refer to *any* deaf person, even those with good speech. Newspapers in the States still use the offensive term "deaf-mute" to refer to deaf persons who communicate in Sign. We urge our readers NOT to use these terms. "Deaf" is simple, accurate, and dignified.

[2] Fanwood is the popular name for the New York School for the Deaf, the second-oldest such school in the United States.

Chapter 27

"Can 'Deaf' be used as a noun (as in 'the Deaf') or should it be used only as an adjective?"

As a librarian actively pursuing increasing both library service to the deaf community and deaf awareness, I find myself walking a tightrope. There is an inconsistency in what people who are deaf expect of hearing people and in regard to vocabulary.

When I first became involved with the deaf community I was told NOT to use deaf as a NOUN. It is an adjective so, of course, we should always say or write "deaf people" or "deaf community." I find that logical and correct, and yet organizations use deaf as a NOUN and actually use hearing as a NOUN too when referring to deaf and hearing people.

Recently I've become aware that a number of individuals don't want to be designated as "deaf artist" or "deaf writer." Rather they are "writers who happen to be deaf." While I can understand this also it's a little difficult to say the above phrase or write it consistently.

I guess physical characteristics are different from ethnic, racial, or religious affiliations but at the same time, we use those both as NOUNS and ADJECTIVES; i.e., "Jews" and "Jewish People."

Anyway, can you help me with my dilemma?

S. L.
Cleveland Heights, Ohio

mong members of a group (e.g., ethnic or religious), certain permissible ("in-group") expressions take on a negative connotation when used by outsiders. Some Deaf people will actually use the word "Deaf" to mean *a Deaf person*: "A group of Deafs traveled to Hawaii." This would be unacceptable usage from a hearing person; it would undoubtedly be construed as an insult. And not all Deaf people like that usage. Likewise, some Deaf persons use the word "Deafie" as a term of affection; other Deaf persons dislike it.

Using "the Deaf" without "people" or "community" is certainly acceptable usage in the Deaf community. Witness: National Theatre of the Deaf; National Association of the Deaf; National Fraternal Society of the Deaf; Telecommunications for the Deaf, Inc.; etcetera. Similar adjectives are often used without their referent word "persons" or "people"; e.g., *The Young and Restless*, "the gifted," "the blind," "the handicapped." Deaf people use "the Hearing"—or even "Hearings"—in the same way. One gets used to it.

It's impossible to formulate hard-and-fast rules about common informal usage. Much depends on the sensibilities of the Deaf persons in question, how strongly they identify with the cultural-Deaf community, how important (or marginal) their deafness is in relation to their work, and how they feel about hearing people using the term "the Deaf." This goes for *Deaf writer* versus *writer who happens to be deaf*. Consider the differences in connotation. Of course, it helps to have some familiarity with the corpus of their work. When in doubt, proceed cautiously.

In conclusion, we'd like to share an anecdote from Richard Nowell, a veteran interpreter, teacher, researcher, administrator, audiologist, and parent coun-

selor who has worked extensively with Deaf performers, and who is currently Associate Professor in "Education of Persons with Hearing Loss" at Indiana University of Pennsylvania. His view is worth noting:

Many years ago when I was still a new professional in the field of
education of persons with hearing loss, I attended a meeting at
Gallaudet. I presented a talk in which I made several references to
"the deaf." After my presentation was finished, a deaf man (I have
no recollection who it was) came up to me and gently signed to me
something like this:

"When you use the term 'the deaf,' you seem to be talking about
us as if we were all the same. That offends many deaf people. It's
better to say something like 'deaf persons' instead of 'the deaf.'"

He didn't act angry with me. He didn't embarrass me in front of
other people. He didn't make me feel bad. He simply taught me an
important lesson in a very constructive way.

Although I won't say that I have never slipped and used the term
"the deaf" since then, I have done my best to avoid it. And after our
conversation, I felt even more strongly that I liked being part of the
Deaf World. There is a right way and a wrong way to teach dumb
hearing people like me this kind of lesson.*

*"I'm Training You to Teach Students Whose Ears Don't Work
Right," the eighth installment of his series "The Way I Hear It. . .,"
DEAF LIFE, December, 1991.

Chapter 28

When I use the word "handicapped," my deaf friends get angry. Why is that?

here are two basic ways to see deafness: as a physical disability or an ethnic difference. The "disability" outlook includes describing deafness as a "communication disorder" or a disease; the "ethnic" outlook sees deaf persons as whole, possessing a distinct language and culture. Needless to say, if *we* believed that being deaf amounted to no more than living under a disability, we wouldn't have started **DEAF LIFE**. Or written this book.

The word "handicap" has an interesting origin: gaming. According to the **American Heritage Dictionary**, it derives from *hand in cap*, "originally a lottery game in which players held forfeits in a cap." It now carries a variety of meanings, primarily the one associated with horse-racing: "a race or contest in which advantages or compensations are given different contestants according to their varied abilities or experience, to equalize the chances of winning." It also means (a) "a deficiency, especially an anatomical, physiological, or mental deficiency, that prevents or restricts normal achievement;" (b) "any disadvantage or disability," and this is the definition we're concerned with. The term "handicapped" is likewise defined as (1) "disabled or crippled;" (2) "mentally deficient;" (3) "having or being under a handicap. Said of a contestant."

Of course, if you consider deafness in purely medical terms, it's a disability; it's a disorder; it's a deficiency; it's a handicap. But suppose that deaf people overwhelmingly rejected this view because they found it too limiting? The majority of deaf people do NOT see themselves as handicapped. As in the famous statement by Dr. I. King Jordan: "Deaf people can do anything . . . except hear." We can't hear? Isn't *that* a disability? By this definition, *everybody* has a disability. Some hearing people can't dance; some have no artistic skill whatsoever; some have lousy coordination; some have no sense of humor; some have poor memories. Yet these same folks would not be eager to let themselves be labeled as "handicapped." Deaf people who dislike being similarly labeled don't like being lumped into one misleading category and dehumanized: "Handicapped? What do you mean? I live a full life. I work; I pay taxes."

The "ethnic" view sees deaf people as different from hearing folks, but just as whole—not merely a set of defective auditory organs. This is a sensible and humane view, although it is not one held by the majority of doctors, specialists, and audiologists—those whose business it is to "fix" what's "wrong" with deaf people's "hearing disorders."

Unfortunately, "handicapped" has acquired a negative connotation. It suggests social inferiority, poverty, hopelessness; it solicits pity, not respect. It makes us shudder. Some deaf people consider it an insult, equivalent to calling a Black person "nigger" or a Hispanic-American "wetback." Not all deaf people object to being called "handicapped." But it's not a bad idea to avoid using the term. Why not simply say "deaf"? If you want to know how *they* feel about the word, ask them directly.

Every person, deaf, hearing, or whatever, is an individual. Let this not be forgotten. We need to get beyond

the limitations imposed by labels. Seeing—*really* seeing—people in terms of something more than a "physical deficiency" isn't just socially courteous, it's politically smart as well.

Chapter 29

Do deaf parents breed deaf children?

his may not sound like a civilized question, but it's certainly one that has been asked many times in many cultures, by supposedly civilized people. And it's still being asked.

There is a philosophy (or pseudo-science) called "eugenics," which deals with inherited characteristics and the possibility of improving (or controlling) those of succeeding generations by "choosing suitable parents." Suitable parents would be encouraged to breed, while unsuitable parents would be discouraged, even prevented, from having "inferior-quality" children. Eugenics was a popular topic in the 19th century, when many hearing educators and philosophers decided that it was better for the "future of the race" if deaf people could be prevented from reproducing more deaf people. Even Alexander Graham Bell, whose own mother and wife were deaf and who invented the telephone while seeking a device to help hard-of-hearing people hear, subscribed to this absurd notion. In his **Memoir Upon the Formation of a Deaf Variety of the Human Race**, he discussed various measures for preventing deaf people from breeding. He proposed legislation to prohibit deaf people from marrying each other, although admitting that this was an impractical expedient.*

However, as a result of the wide publicity given to Bell's theories. a number of American deaf children were sterilized. During the early years of the German Third Reich, the Nazis carried this practice even further, forcibly sterilizing many deaf Jewish and Christian schoolchildren and young adults to ensure that they would never be able to breed "defectives."

What are the facts? Simply this: 90% of all deaf people have hearing parents. And 90% of all deaf parents have hearing children. The facts speak for themselves. Anyone who wants to prevent deaf babies from being born should prevent hearing people from breeding.

In earlier generations, some tyrannical parents tried to prevent their deaf children from marrying, unwilling to have them transmit deafness. This was not only cruel but futile. Most "deaf genes" are transmitted by, and inherited from, hearing parents. Furthermore, the genetic tendency towards deafness is a tad unpredictable. The same mother and father may have several hearing children and several deaf, or all deaf, or all hearing, or all hearing but one, or all deaf but one.

Deafness runs congenitally in only a small percentage of families. The genes causing hereditary deafness may be transmitted through hearing persons for generations before they "express" themselves. Even babies who are born deaf may not have inherited their deafness genetically; they may have been prenatally deafened as a result of exposure to the rubella virus, for example. Early-deafened children may have gotten their deafness from a virus (e.g., spinal meningitis), high fever, or accident. Those deafened by exposure to a virus, illness, or accident would not necessarily be carrying any deaf gene whatsoever—even if one or both parents *are* deaf.

The odds are therefore against a deaf parent having a deaf child. But for a deaf child to be born into a deaf family is no tragedy. Indeed, it can be a blessing. What Bell and many others never recognized (much less appreciated) was the quality of life in Deaf surroundings. Far from being "defectives," many Deaf families have enjoyed rich, fulfilling lives. Most Deaf parents who have deaf children immediately accept them as normal children (something a good number of hearing parents must struggle to accomplish). To Deaf parents, deafness *is* normal. There's nothing wrong, bad, inferior, or defective about it. Since so many Deaf parents are fluent Signers, deaf children born into such families begin life with complete immersion in the language of the parents. The communication barrier, so common in hearing families with deaf children, simply doesn't exist. So deaf children of Deaf parents start school with a considerable advantage over deaf children from nonsigning hearing families.

Deaf children of Deaf parents have traditionally been the transmitters of sign language and Deaf culture to their schoolmates; the leaders, the boat-rockers. They tend to grow up with a sense of identity, a pride that many deaf children of hearing parents initially lack. Paternalistic hearing people do not take kindly to the idea of dynasties of uppity Deaf folks. Few of our oppressors have ever sought the truth beneath the invidious stereotype.

The quality of parenting, not the health of the auditory nerves, is what's important. To make a general statement: since many Deaf parents have positive feelings about their own deafness, they are correspondingly more accepting of others' deafness, and transmit those feelings to their own deaf children, who grow up with a positive self-image, a more comfortable sense of identity than many deaf children of hearing parents. As noted above, that's a definite advantage. Deaf parents can offer what any good parent does: acceptance, love, patience, wisdom, morality, and guidance towards eventual independence.

*See also Chapters 38 and 39.

Chapter 30

Do all deaf people benefit from hearing aids?

o. A hearing aid is not a miracle machine. It's a tiny amplifier. It makes sounds louder, and that's all it can do. It amplifies everything it picks up, without distinction—all sounds that happen to pop up in the immediate area as well as distracting background noises like traffic. A hearing aid cannot "zero in" on the voice or voices you most want to pick up; it doesn't work selectively, as our hearing does. And it cannot make other people's speech clearer, merely a bit louder. So if a speaker's articulation is not particularly good—for example, if he's a mumbler—or if his face is not clearly visible, a hearing aid is of very little help.

Because even severely deaf persons have some degree of recognition of certain sounds, many do wear powerful hearing aids to pick up whatever sounds they can; they feel it helps make them more aware of what's going on. Others do not feel comfortable with an aid and don't like to wear them. Many Deaf people function quite well without any electronic doojizmos.

How does a deaf person decide whether or not to wear an aid? As part of "early intervention," even newborns can be fitted with aids. The tendency has been to fit young deaf children, even profoundly deaf ones, with aids, especially in mainstreamed schools. This decision is made by the parents, educators, and audiologists who want the child to be "as normal as possible." The child's own feelings have seldom, if ever, been taken into account. The implication is that a hearing aid gives a deaf child a semblance of normality—makes him or her more like a Hearing child, more part of the Hearing world. Often, the actual benefits of wearing an aid (if there are any) are far outweighed by the sheer discomfort. Not surprisingly, some of these children grow up with bitter memories of being forced to wear bulky body-pack aids, enduring the discomfort, even pain, of being plugged into a machine that amplified gibberish. (Ironically, repeated exposure to loud amplification can damage the residual hearing—the very residual hearing that audiologists are striving to protect!) Children with this kind of background are understandably resentful and unenthusiastic about wearing aids. No Deaf child or adult should ever be forced to wear a hearing aid.

As for residential schools, most deaf children are encouraged to wear aids, but some enlightened professionals recognize that even heavy amplification isn't really going to benefit some kids. Some parents let the children decide for themselves. Some kids who fight the aid when they're young choose to wear one when they're older. By the time a child is old enough to leave home and set off for college, work, or whatever, she can decide whether to continue wearing an aid.

Adults who feel that an aid might help them can get tested by an audiologist, and try some of the many aids on the market before choosing the one that's best for their needs. Expense, of course, is a consideration. Hearing aids are exorbitantly costly.

Some Deaf people, we've noticed, wear aids all the time—even when they're with other Deaf people who Sign fluently! Others wear them when they want to listen to a concert or something of special interest on TV, or to use a telephone or an audio loop in a theater. Others never wear them. It's a matter of personal preference.

▲ ▲ ▲

The Cochlear-Implant Controversy

In the summer of 1990, the U.S. Food and Drug Administration approved cochlear implants for children aged 2-17. Previously, only adults had been able to get implants. Now the green light was given to implanting children without their consent.

A cochlear implant is a "bionic ear" device. A small receiver is implanted in the mastoid bone behind the ear; an array of electrodes (22 for the 22-channel device) is inserted surgically into the cochlea (the snail-shaped organ of the inner ear). This operation involves drilling a hole in the skull. After one month of healing, the implantee is fitted with an ear-level microphone and a transmitting coil attached by a cord to a speech processor, a sort of pocket computer. The microphone picks up sounds, relays them to the speech processor, which transmits them to the receiver behind the ear, which sends the signals to the internal device, which stimulates the auditory nerve, which sends these signals to the brain, which interprets them as "sounds."

Candidates for implants are those who have little or no usable hearing in one or both ears. A cochlear implant does NOT completely restore hearing to the implanted ear, nor is the quality of sound completely "natural." An implantee, ideally, will be able to hear a wider variety of sounds and develop better speech patterns. They may or may not be able to use the telephone.

The long-range effects of such a device are unknown. What sort of effect the constant electronic stimulation may have on the tissue and nerves of the inner ear is likewise unknown. Many deaf people feel that this is a rather drastic expedient. Hearing aids, vibrotactile devices, auditory trainers, and FM systems are at least removable. A cochlear implant is there to stay.

Results have been mixed. While some children and adults certainly benefit from an implant, others have benefited very little. In a few cases, the results have been horrible—the body painfully rejects the implant, or the implant destroys whatever residual hearing there was. It's impossible to predict if an implant will be accepted and will benefit the implantee. The implantee may enjoy considerable improvement in the quality of sound, or moderate, or practically none.

Needless to say, cochlear implants are fantastically expensive, and the companies who manufacture them tout their benefits. They claim that a child with an implant will have more options and better social, educational, and job opportunities. It's estimated that no more than 1% of the deaf population are good candidates for implants, yet those who support its use are enthusiastic about the possibility of wiping out deafness—making it "obsolete."

The Deaf community is certainly not against adults voluntarily undergoing the operation and receiving implants. Late-deafened adults often make excellent candidates. For example, a number of ALDAns (members of the Association of Late-Deafened Adults) have received implants, and love them. A few have gotten mediocre results, and a very few have had bad results.

Deaf-rights advocates tried, but were unable, to prevent the FDA from approving implants for children. Many of us were disturbed by the FDA's decision. Why?

For one thing, Deaf people themselves—deaf children grown up—have had no say in the matter. Their views, and their real concern for other deaf children, formed by long and hard first-hand experience, are typically dismissed as irrelevant by those who have the power—the hearing oralists, scientists, executives, audiologists, and governmental officials.

We feel that deaf children should be exposed to sign language as well as speech, as part of a Total Communication or Bilingual-Bicultural curriculum. They can choose whatever mode they feel most comfortable with. They can elect to wear a hearing aid, and when they're old enough, voluntarily receive an implant. Or not. The issue is choice. Some Deaf people feel that it's a decision ONLY deaf people can make for themselves. Others feel that implants should be outlawed, period.

An implant is the ultimate invasion of the ear, the ultimate denial of deafness, the ultimate refusal to let deaf children be Deaf. Those who make the decision to implant children choose to risk the children's health so that they can hear more sounds and develop clearer speech. Children attending oral schools and mainstream programs are the most likely to be implanted. Their parents, the ones who choose to have their children implanted, are in effect saying, "I don't respect the Deaf community, and I certainly don't want my child to be part of it. I want him/her to be part of the hearing world, not the Deaf world."

Chapter 31

Why do most deaf parents raise a hearing child better than hearing parents a deaf child?
(If you cannot answer or agree, may a tribe of your researchers increase!)

"Avid Reader"
Jackson, Mississippi

s with so many other aspects of the Deaf reality, it all depends on the individual—in this case, the parents and the child.

Hearing children of hearing parents begin communicating by babbling, then making recognizable words, then forming complete sentences, expanding their vocabularies daily. By listening, they absorb spoken language effortlessly, unconsciously. And they learn by imitating others—in this case, their parents, who give them constant feedback, correcting mispronunciations and grammatical errors. Hearing children of deaf parents often lack this vital auditory/oral feedback process. Since so many deaf adults don't use their voices, or have unnatural-sounding voices even if they *do* speak, their children often don't pick up good speech patterns—clear articulation, intonation, and expression. They tend to develop poor early speech patterns. Many require speech therapy once they start school.

Much depends on the home environment—how intellectual it is, and whether or not a hearing child of deaf parents has access to other hearing children, relatives, and family friends, who can act as good "speech models." Consider a hearing child of deaf parents who live on a farm. Their nearest neighbors may be miles away. These children would have little or no early exposure to spoken language, and, conversely, far less opportunity to develop good oral skills. (Having a radio or TV helps, but they're no substitute for real face-to-face interaction.) A hearing child of deaf parents in a friendly, well-populated town or urban neighborhood would undoubtedly have an easier time of it.

Some deaf parents are simply indifferent to their children's communication needs. They need exposure to speech? Too bad. Let them get it somewhere else. (Some deaf children of hearing parents are likewise stuck in a deprived environment.)

Preschoolers are routinely tested for language skills. Unfortunately, this puts many hearing children of deaf parents at an immediate disadvantage. They are often labeled "language-deficient" because ASL, not English, is their first language. They're in roughly the same pickle as Spanish-speaking children who get similarly labeled. They may be absolutely fluent in their native language, but that skill doesn't count in an English-speaking environment.

Needless to say, most deaf parents (a good 90%) are aware of the problem, concerned about their children's well-being, and do something about it. They want to know where to go, what they can do, where to get help. They ask questions, call the schools, and try to find preschool programs that can benefit their children.

Hearing children of Deaf parents, of course, do have a native language, which puts them ahead of deaf children of hearing parents who can't communicate effectively with them. (Such children often start school without any language at all.) However, they tend to lag behind hearing children of hearing parents, who already have an advantage in spoken-language skills and socialization. Nonetheless, with proper speech training and classroom support, hearing children of deaf parents will do fine. They'll catch up, and sometimes surpass their classmates.

All deaf Americans are, to a lesser or greater extent, bilingual. They are surrounded by "Hearing"-American-English-language culture. They cannot help absorbing it. (In the case of English, sometimes forcibly.) Consequently, they tend to understand the demands of the Hearing world far better than the Hearing world understands their needs as Deaf people. Involved in a "mixed" conversation, they will go to great lengths to make sure the hearing person understands them. (They will "switch codes" from ASL to Pidgin Sign English, fingerspell, speak, write, use body language, or a combination of modes.) They are sensitized to the need for accessible communication. Their experience as members of a Deaf community and a Hearing society gives them a dual perspective. Ideally, they *can* do a fine job of raising their children, deaf or hearing, as bilingual citizens.

It's foolish to make sweeping generalizations about hearing children of deaf parents, but for some, the bilingual-bicultural orientation obviously influences them in their choice of careers. Many become interpreters. Others become teachers and educators, linguists, researchers, social workers, service providers, performers, or writers. Many enjoy their connection to the Deaf community and remain fluent signers.

No doubt, a tribe of researchers are undertaking studies right now to determine just how hearing children of Deaf parents learn, and what effect the early exposure to ASL may have on their language development.

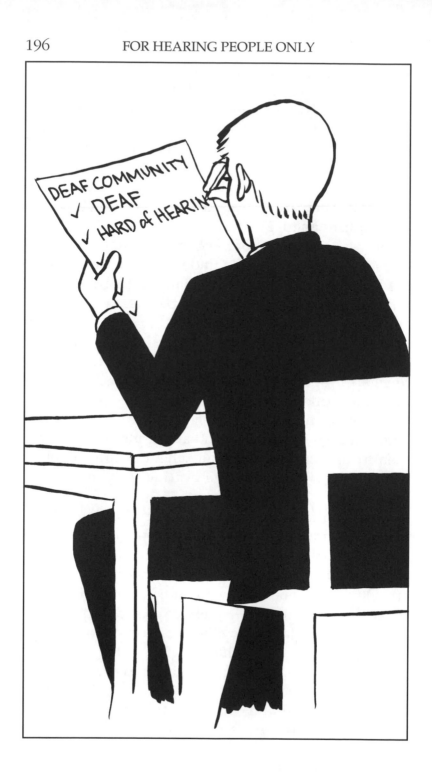

Chapter 32

I know that the Deaf community includes both "deaf" and "hard-of-hearing." What other categories are there?

he term "Deaf community" can be broadly applied to include all those in the "hearing-loss" end of the spectrum. This includes those deaf from birth ("congenitally deaf"), those who become deaf very early in life ("pre-lingually deaf"), those deafened later in life ("adventitiously deaf"), as well as late-deafened adults, and hard-of-hearing persons of all ages. People who suffer from tinnitus, a disorder causing unnatural noises—buzzing, ringing, clicking, roaring—in the ears, should also be included, as tinnitus is a form of hearing impairment. The same for those with Ménière's disease, a more severe progressive inner-ear disorder that includes attacks of tinnitus and vertigo (extreme dizziness).

Some audiologically hard-of-hearing people are culturally Deaf and function as Deaf people. But some audiologically deaf people prefer to function (and identify themselves) as hard-of-hearing and remain within the Hearing world. This, of course, does not rule out having a good relationship with the Deaf community!

Then there are audiologically deaf (deafened) people who are struggling through an identity crisis. They stubbornly deny that they're deaf; they insist that they're "hard-of-hearing." We know of a progressively deafened woman who is angry. She wants to be "hard-of-hearing," not "deaf." But she *is* deaf. She's angry because she can't be a part of the Hearing world any more, and doesn't *want* to be a part of the Deaf world. Not yet, anyway. Her speech pathologist feels that learning Sign would be good for her. But for some late-deafened people, that's too drastic, too uncomfortable a step. Hearing loss, especially the sudden kind, can be exceedingly difficult to cope with; it can be devastating, even life-threatening. Let no one underestimate it.

The Deaf community ideally includes those who are culturally Deaf—native and longtime ASL users—as well as those who are deaf but are oriented towards oral means of communication—auditory aids, speechreading and cued speech. Many culturally Deaf people wear hearing aids; some don't. There are radical differences between the needs of the culturally Deaf and the needs of the late-deafened, the progressively deaf, and the hard-of-hearing. Yet all share the same concerns—the need for support services, fair treatment, and accessible communication.

Moreover, the Deaf community includes a number of hearing people: parents and relatives of deaf children; friends, families, and spouses of deaf adults; supporters and advocates; some teachers, administrators, professionals, and service providers. They respect Deaf people and have earned the respect of the Deaf community.

Categorizing *can* easily become an exercise in absurdity. But the basic needs of the Deaf community as a whole, whatever "category" each member can be placed in, are clear enough: unrestricted communication and unrestricted access to everything hearing people benefit from and take for granted—TV programming, education, government offices, public-service agencies, public announcements, hospitals, business networks—*right down to the totals on supermarket cash registers*. That means visual (or audio-visual) aids, sensitive architectural design, captioning, interpreters (whether sign-language or oral), better telephone relay services, more public TTYs,* and, equally important, more public awareness. There's still far too little.

The Americans with Disabilities Act went into effect January 26, 1992. It prohibits discrimination on the basis of disability in public accommodations, transportation, etc. The ADA includes deaf and hard-of-hearing persons. It is too soon to tell what sort of permanent impact it will have on the Deaf community. But things are astir. The first ADA lawsuits on behalf of Deaf plaintiffs have already been filed.

As long as Deaf people are discriminated against in schooling, employment, social and civil rights, as long as they are seen as "strange" and "different" and "second-class," they will protest, make themselves seen—and heard. All members of the Deaf community, as U.S. citizens, have specific needs, and our democratic society is obligated to ensure that those needs are met.

---

*A TTY (teletypewriter or Teletype machine) is also known as a TDD (telecommunication device for the deaf). The newest terms, adding still more confusion to the alphabet soup, are TT, TTP, or TexTel (all standing for "text telephone").

Chapter 33

What are some of the biggest problems faced by late-deafened people?

late-deafened adult is generally defined as someone who became deaf—whether progressively, suddenly, or even genetically—after age 18. As a rule, the later the age at the onset of deafness, the more difficult the adjustment. Those who become deaf as teenagers will have a relatively easier time than those in their 20's or 30's or 40's—which is not to say that adjustment is easy for *anyone*; it's not. But a younger person will usually find it easier to cope than someone with an established career, marriage, children, and a stable pattern of life. Teens have a certain amount of fluidity and instability in their lives, and this can be an advantage. The more established the patterns, the more painful the unraveling.

Late-deafened people, as hearing persons who have recently lost or are progressively losing their hearing, have a more complicated time of it than those born deaf or early-deafened. To some extent, they can choose how deeply they want to remain involved in the Hearing world and enter the Deaf world—but they cannot function as "normal" hearing people anymore. They grapple with the realization that they can no longer enjoy certain "ordinary" things hearing people take for granted—picking up a telephone and making a whispered call, music, conversations, family dinners, interacting with children and grandchildren, chit-chat and jokes, on-the-job communication, the everyday heard and spoken details of life. Virtually everything familiar and comfortable in their lives, the foundation of their very sanity, is shaken. A late-deafened person sees his or her identity coming undone, dissolving without any "resolving" in sight. It's not something that's solved by simply buying a TTY or enrolling in a "Basic Sign Communication" class. It can be devastating.

Late-deafness strikes at the very heart of relationships: the ability to communicate freely and openly with each other, to understand and to be understood. One tragic consequence is the breakup not just of friendships, but of families. A number of "rock-solid" marriages have fallen apart when one partner becomes deaf. Late-deafened workers sometimes lose their jobs. Isolation, depression, and suicidal impulses are the most dangerous result of this process. You're not hearing any more, and you're not culturally Deaf, so where do you fit in? What sort of future can there be?

One of the worst aspects of being late-deafened is the incomprehension of "well-meaning" relatives and friends, and the horrendous things that are said in the guise of "consolation." A prime example: the obnoxious sentence, "You have to learn to accept your deafness." "Deafness" here has a decidedly negative connotation: Accept the fact that you're an auditory cripple. Accept the fact that you have to settle for an inferior form of existence. Accept the fact that your social life is kaput. Accept isolation. Accept *what*? Losing one's hearing is not necessarily the end of the world, but "advice" like this, intended to assuage grief, makes things worse. Hearing people say things like this to cover their own feelings of embarrassment. Or, perhaps, their utter inadequacy.

The Deaf community has many things that are good about it, and many things that are bad—such as a kind

of quasi clannish, insular snobbishness. Some late-deafened people, eager to reach out to and be accepted by the
Deaf community, bravely venture into new territory—
a Deaf gathering—only to find themselves getting the
frozen-shoulder treatment. They're viewed as "hear-
ings-in-the-head," and accorded the coldest imaginable
welcome, which is no welcome at all. To be fair, not all
Deaf people greet "newcomers" with hostile rejection,
but many do, and it's enough to scare anyone off. Thus,
the people in greatest need of understanding and support from this community are often treated with cruelty.
And this is a terrible injustice.

Late-deafened people find their greatest support from
each other—those who have experienced the forcible
severance from the hearing world, and survived. That's
why the Association of Late-Deafened Adults (ALDA)
was founded, and that's the key to its considerable
success. Networking. It's important for late-deafened
people to know that they're *not* alone, and that their
problems are real, not figments of their tormented minds.
And many of these problems *do* have solutions.

Chapter 34

How do people become deaf?

 e're either born deaf or become deaf. A person born deaf is said to be *congenitally deaf*; a person who becomes deaf after birth is *adventitiously deaf*. Adventitious deafness can be either *pre-lingual* (occurring during the first 3 years of life), or *post-lingual* (becoming deaf after age 3). And the area of post-lingual deafness is further subdivided into *childhood deafness, pre-vocational deafness* (becoming deaf while still a teenager), or *post-vocational deafness* (becoming deaf while an adult). A "deafened adult" is one who became deaf after age 19. One can also be described as "early-deafened" or "late-deafened." Interestingly, more males than females are early-deafened, but since women tend to outlive men, there are more late-deafened elderly women than men.

What does all this fancy terminology mean? Many Deaf people (i.e., those with a strong cultural affiliation to the Signing Deaf community) are congenitally deaf or early-deafened. Deafness that runs in the family (*genetically transmitted, hereditary,* or *inherited deafness*) is a relatively rare cause. More common is prenatal exposure to a virus. The rubella (German measles) epidemic of the mid-1960s affected many pregnant women whose children were subsequently born deaf. The Rh factor and prematurity are two other causes of congenital deafness. When no specific cause can be determined, one's deafness is described as "of unknown etiology." This handy phrase crops up in the medical histories of a large number of deaf people.

It should be noted that *congenital* and *hereditary* deafness are *not* synonymous. Congenitally deaf means born deaf. But not all congenitally deaf people have hereditary deafness. Children born deaf because of prenatal exposure to the rubella virus may not be carrying any gene whatsoever for deafness. Conversely, someone who has hereditary deafness may be born with normal hearing that progressively deteriorates—and the cause is pinpointed as hereditary.

Adventitious deafness can be caused by accidents (as when I. King Jordan, the first deaf president of Gallaudet University, was hurled off his motorcycle), bomb blasts, injuries (e.g., punctured eardrums) extreme chill, high fever, viral infections such as mumps, meningitis, and encephalitis, diseases such as neurofibromatosis-2 (tumors that attack the auditory nerves), and reactions to certain (ototoxic) drugs.

Gradual hearing loss can result from repeated doses of very deep or high noise—e.g., blasting-loud rock concerts, commuting on the subway, constant exposure to industrial hazards such as operating a pneumatic drill, or even living too near an airport. Otosclerosis—hardening of the bones of the middle ear—is common among older people. There are numerous causes of deafness, and you're likely to meet deaf persons from a wide variety of "backgrounds." There is no blanket definition of deafness; all deaf persons are individuals.

Often a Deaf person will greet a stranger by asking "Are you Deaf?—were you born deaf?" That's their way of "sounding out" the new person—getting a quick idea of their ethnic identity, so to speak—their background, outlook, and place in the Deaf community.

Deaf Awareness: 5-Minute Quiz

Chapters 26—34

Answers are on the bottom of the page, upside down.

True or False:

1. The vast majority of deaf people have perfectly normal vocal apparatus. Those who don't talk choose not to because they don't feel comfortable using their voices, not because they *can't* talk.

2. Most deaf people consider themselves handicapped.

3. The majority of deaf people have deaf parents.

4. Late-deafened people have traditionally been eagerly accepted into the Deaf community and accorded a warm welcome.

5. *Congenital* and *hereditary* deafness are the same thing.

Chapter 35

"Is hearing loss common in my family because of heredity, or because my grandmother fell down during her pregnancies?"

I have been reading some articles of "For Hearing People Only" and noticed if someone has questions, to write for information.

I have an uncle and aunt who are brother and sister; they are both deaf. Their mother, my grandmother, is deaf in one ear. My aunt has a daughter who is deaf in one ear and my uncle has a daughter who has some hearing loss in both ears. I have been diagnosed with Meniere's Disease.[1] I am curious to know if it is possible for all this hearing loss to be hereditary in my family as it is quite ironic. My uncle and aunt were both born deaf, and the doctor told my grandparents that the reason why they are deaf is because my grandmother fell down during both pregnancies. Is this just an explanation due to lack of knowledge or is this possible?

If you can't answer [this question,] I understand; I thought I would inquire anyway.

S.M.
Sydney, Nova Scotia

t looks as though your family carries a genetic tendency towards hearing loss, deafness, and hearing disorders. Assuming one gene is responsible (and there may be a number of them), it "expresses" itself (shows up) to different degrees among different members of your family; more females than males seem to be affected. It is not *that* uncommon for deafness and hearing disorders (possibly including Ménière's disease) to run in families. One of our staffers is congenitally and genetically deaf. Although his mother is hearing, she was a carrier of the gene for deafness, as (hereditary) deafness ran in her family. One of her two sons was born deaf, the other hearing. It's like the genetic tendencies toward nearsightedness (myopia), color-blindness, diabetes, or obesity. Some 10% of deaf people have deaf parents. So "deafness" genes are mostly carried throughout the hearing population.

There is much we don't yet understand about genetics. But we'd wager that babies are **NOT** born deaf because their mothers fell down during their pregnancies! Your grandmother's doctor was absolutely mistaken. We're sure of it. Why? A simple medical fact: the fetus floats weightlessly, completely surrounded by fluid, in the amniotic sac—a great shock absorber—further protected by the mother's body *and* the layers of clothing she will undoubtedly be wearing (unless she slips in the bathtub!).

We consulted a veteran nurse-midwife, and she assured us that if a woman suffers a fall during pregnancy, *she* may hurt, but the fetus will, in all likelihood, be absolutely safe. If a pregnant woman suffers a bad fall, she *may* have a miscarriage. But in most cases, she will carry the pregnancy safely to term; the baby will be born healthy. (In many instances miscarriages are spontaneous, unconnected with a fall or injury; there is something wrong with the embryo and the body expels it.)

And *if* the mother's fall *were* to injure the fetus, why would it affect only the baby's inner ears? It would seem more logical for a baby injured before birth to be born with dislocated limbs or major injuries, not defective hearing. It also seems quite improbable that falls during two different pregnancies would result in the exact same thing: deafness. Now, assuming that your grandmother *did* fall during both pregnancies, it's possible that her falls were the result of a balance problem which was itself hereditary. In other words, the same hereditary inner-ear problem could have caused your grandmother to feel dizzy, lose her balance, and fall, *and then* showed up in her children as well. There's no sense blaming the poor woman for falls which may or may not have happened. It's pretty obviously a genetic problem, and there is a simple genetic explanation.

In the days when very few people understood much, if anything, about heredity, folklore ascribed all manner of birth defects and disabilities to the mother's misdeeds or mishaps: children born with cleft palates, for example, were thought to result from a hare's running across the mother's path while she was pregnant.[2] Such beliefs caused the unfortunate mothers (as well as the children) tremendous guilt, pain, and shame. It's easy to say that the doctor should have known better; this was only a couple of generations ago. But genetic research is a relatively new field, and old presumptions die hard.

If you or your relatives are curious or concerned about the possibility of transmitting deafness to your children, we recommend you see a genetic counselor, who can test you, give you a more informed idea of the odds, and provide reassurance.

[1] Ménière's disease is "an inner-ear disorder of unknown origin that causes hearing loss, dizziness or vertigo and tinnitus (noises within the head). [It] affects more than one million Americans and can be extremely incapacitating." (Carol Turkington and Allen E. Sussman, Ph.D., eds., **The Encyclopedia of Deafness and Hearing Disorders**, pp. 121-122.)

[2] Even more dire is the old English folk belief that it was the *devil* in the form of a hare. So both mother and child were in league with the devil—accursed. (See next chapter.)

Chapter 36

Is deafness "bad karma"?

oughly speaking, *karma* (or *karman*) means effects, fate or destiny. Hinduism and Buddhism, for example, teach that a soul is born and reborn many times, in different forms. **The American Heritage Dictionary** defines karma as "the sum and consequences of a person's actions during the successive phases of his existence, regarded as determining his destiny." The **Longman Dictionary of Contemporary English** defines it a bit more simply as "the force produced by a person's actions in one life on earth which will influence his [or her] next life on earth." In other words, what you do in this life will have an effect on your next life. This has led to the tragic belief that a deaf or disabled person must have done something bad in a previous life to deserve the punishment of being born "defective."

The idea of being "cursed" is by no means limited to Hindus or Buddhists. In ancient Greece, fathers had the right to abandon "defective" babies, who were taken in baskets to the mountains and left to die of exposure.[1] While the Torah carries an explicit prohibition against cursing the deaf,[2] the New Testament has a decidedly negative view. The few deaf persons mentioned in the gospels are described as possessed by an evil spirit.[3]

According to the Jewish Scriptures (a.k.a. "the Old Testament"), God created deaf people as part of a divine plan. But the New Testament view stuck. For thousands of years in Christian Europe, deaf people were considered not fully human, incapable of learning, and unworthy of salvation. This attitude survives today, for example, in certain Latin American countries. Even in the United States, there is a widespread belief that God punishes parents through their children. Some people honestly believe that children are born disabled because their parents did something evil.

The belief in reincarnation (or "transmigration of souls") is not limited to Hinduism or Buddhism, either. Plato accepted it (the Greek term is *metempsychosis*). Judaism certainly accepts it—the Hebrew term is *gilgul nefesh*, the "rolling" or "recycling" of a soul.

If you wish to take a mystical approach, you can look at karma (or reincarnation) either negatively or positively. In the negative interpretation, a soul is born as a deaf person as a punishment—i.e., bad karma. But according to the positive interpretation, a soul chooses to be born as a deaf person as a challenge or learning experience. The Deaf soul experiences the restrictions, prejudices, and hostilities of the hearing world so that it may progress to a higher level of spiritual understanding. This in no way contradicts the doctrine of free will— that whatever our station in life, we have the freedom to choose how we respond to it. The ultimate challenge is to choose wisely.[4]

---

[1] As in Sophocles' classic Greek tragedy, **Oedipus**. Laius, king of Thebes, husband of Queen Jocasta, is warned by an oracle that his newborn son will slay him. He tries to forestall this by abandoning the baby to certain death on Mount Cithaeron—pinning the baby's heels together and stringing him up on a tree-branch. The baby is rescued by a compassionate shepherd, and Oedipus ("swollen foot" or "wounded heel" or) survives, and ultimately fulfills the prophecy, killing his father, becoming king of Thebes, and marrying his own mother, Jocasta.

[2] Leviticus 19:14: "You shall not curse the deaf, nor put a stumbling-block before the blind." However, in Jewish law, deaf persons were considered "legally incompetent," whether or not they could communicate via writing. If you could not speak—i.e., were

a *kheresh* ("deaf-mute")—you were not legally competent. Deaf-mutes (along with idiots, minors, slaves, and women) were considered legally incompetent by the majority of rabbinic authorities, capable by some. For a man, "legally incompetent" meant, for example, being disqualified from serving as a witness in a rabbinical court or being counted in a *minyan* (prayer quorum). (All women, hearing or deaf, were automatically barred from these privileges.) But the social reality was complex. Deaf Jews could earn a living, study Torah, and (in some cases) marry.

3 In the Gospel of St. Mark, for example, a father brings his deaf-mute son to Jesus, after the disciples were unable to cure him. The "dumb spirit" frequently throws the boy into violent convulsions; he foams at the mouth, grinds his teeth, and "pines away." Jesus exorcises the "dumb and deaf spirit":

> And when Jesus saw that a crowd came running together, he rebuked the unclean spirit, saying to it, "You dumb and deaf spirit, I command you, come out of him, and never enter him again."
> [Afterwards,] his disciples asked him privately, "Why could we not cast it out?" And he said to them, "This kind cannot be driven out by anything but prayer."
> (Mark 9:14-29; **The New Oxford Annotated Bible**, Revised Standard Version, 1973)

As Attorney Paulette Caswell points out, the boy seems to be an epileptic. For a long time, epileptics were considered "idiots" and "incompetents" in the eyes of the law. This attitude probably developed from the early Christian belief that they were possessed by "evil spirits." In the New Testament, deaf-mutes have not only a physical disability, but mental and spiritual ones as well. See "In the Eyes of the Law, Are We (Really) Equal?", **DEAF LIFE**, March 1992.

4 As originally published in **DEAF LIFE**, this chapter was one of two that provoked strong complaints from readers. Two readers objected to the statement in Chapter 50 about interpreters being seen as people who "earn money off Deaf people's language." One of these two, an Episcopal minister, also argued that the New Testament was simply reflecting the prevalent social attitudes of its time, and that Jesus, in approaching and healing the sick and disabled, who were considered outcasts, was working against these prejudices. Our response was that although both Jewish and Christian traditions have many admirable and positive elements, neither is free of negative attitudes towards deaf people.

Chapter 37

"What is Deaf culture? Has anyone studied it from a sociological perspective?"

From the executive director of a Canadian agency serving Deaf and hard-of-hearing people:

Although we have many books and articles by deaf authors, I have not found a thorough description of Deaf Culture in one book or article. Many people ask our Deaf staff and Board members but it is too big a topic to get an easy answer to "what is Deaf culture?" We are a young and growing agency and we have several staff who are not familiar with Deaf Culture. Do you know of or have a good book, or brochure, that we could order and have available for those who are interested? Has anyone studied Deaf culture from a sociological perspective?

L. E.
Victoria, British Columbia

ne possible definition of U.S. Deaf culture (and there must be many!) is: a social, communal, and creative force of, by, and for Deaf people based on American Sign Language (ASL). It encompasses communication, social protocol, art, entertainment, recreation (e.g., sports, travel, and Deaf clubs), and (to a point) worship. It's also an attitude, and, as such, can be a weapon of prejudice—"You're not one of us; you don't *belong.*"

Despite the mighty efforts of generations of oralists, deaf people still prefer to communicate and mingle with their own kind. That is the psychosocial basis of Deaf culture. Deaf people in the United States have staunchly resisted the efforts of oralists to abolish the use of sign language and assimilate them into the hearing mainstream. The simple fact is that deaf people who attend the common residential schools for the deaf—no matter what mode of communication is forced on them in the classrooms—tend to seek out other deaf people and communicate in sign language. This is true, to some extent, in other countries, but the U.S. arguably has the most sophisticated and creative—and public—Deaf culture of any. As such, it has been quite influential. Think of the internationally acclaimed National Theatre of the Deaf, which is an indirect offshoot of "community" institutions such as the Gallaudet Dramatics Club and Deaf-club productions.

Very broadly speaking, the people who adhere to the Deaf-culture view have attended schools for the deaf, where they picked up ASL from each other and developed a distinctly "Deaf" attitude, encompassing such things as outlook (there is, unfortunately, a certain anti-intellectual bias, a clannish snobbery); sharing information through gossip; teasing and joke-playing; visual humor; and a passion for sports. Certain team sports, notably volleyball, bowling, and basketball, are "Deaf tribal sports." In Deaf tribal sports, *everyone* gets a chance to participate. To Deaf people, sports are a social thing, a kinetic way of expressing "belonging."

Not all Deaf people are fond of the old cultural institution, the Deaf club. These establishments used to perform a vital social function. Deaf people, excluded from the inaccessible medium of the radio, could get together there to share news, information, entertainment (subtitled foreign films and live ASL performances), or simply relax after work, gossip, and enjoy each others' company. (Which is not to say that these clubs were democratic. For many years, some clubs barred women or excluded them from holding office. In keeping with social and educational "norms," some were undoubtedly racially segregated as well—whites and blacks having separate clubs.) With the advent of captioned TV and home videos, the Deaf club has (in some instances) dwindled into a place where Deaf people go to watch videos and gossip. Some clubs have managed to survive, maintaining a high level of sophistication; some don't even have bars.

Some Deaf people do not believe that we have a full-fledged culture in the sense that Blacks, Jews, Italians, (Native) American Indians, or Hispanics have. Ethnic culture is generally transmitted from parent to child, with grandparents and other elders playing important roles. Most Deaf people, however, are born into hearing families; many hearing parents cannot even communicate with their own deaf children. In families where deafness runs congenitally, there tends to be a much stronger identification with Deaf culture—a powerful feeling of Deaf pride. Deaf children of Deaf parents tend to become the leaders in their schools—they are the ones who teach the other kids ASL.

Deaf people are not immediately recognizable as belonging to the Deaf culture in the same way that, say, an Amish woman or man is immediately recognizable as "Amish." In contrast to most other full-fledged cultures, there is no distinct mode of dress, no special cuisine, and no uniquely "Deaf religion," although there are Deaf congregations and Deaf churches. These employ ASL (and some Deaf priests or ministers) in their services, but are largely offshoots of established ministries—

Catholic, Lutheran, or Southern Baptist. Deaf Americans look, act, eat, and worship as other Americans do. The only truly distinctive aspect, the one thing that provides the framework and the cohesion, is ASL. Therefore, some folks prefer to classify "Deaf culture" as a subculture.

A major problem with trying to "track down" a definition of Deaf culture is that it's a relatively new concept. Broadly speaking, the idea of a separate and distinct ASL-based culture as a source of public pride arose during the civil-rights-activism era of the 1960s. Previously, Deaf folks may have been proud of their language, clubs, and dramatic productions, but they were very shy about being seen Signing in public. They were, to some extent, made to feel ashamed and inferior. (It was a hearing linguist, William Stokoe, who finally recognized that ASL was, indeed, a full-fledged language. He was not enthusiastically received at first, not even by the Deaf community.)

"Deaf culture" as a conscious force is still in its early stages, creatively ever-changing, ever-evolving. Deaf people have long been involved in visual arts (painting, sculpture, design, etc.). A new "visual literature" live and on videotape is being produced—ASL poetry, plays, storytelling, humor, folklore, songs, sign-mime—and it's exciting to watch it unfold.

Several of the books listed in our bibliography illuminate and define, to some extent, Deaf culture. A prime resource is Carol Padden and Tom Humphries' **Deaf in America: Voices from a Culture** (1988). The authors are themselves Deaf—a notable exception to the old saw (no longer accurate) that all books about Deaf culture are written by hearing people.

Deaf culture has indeed been studied from a sociological perspective, but the old theories are in need of revision.[1] There are some useful published works— Paul C. Higgins' book **Outsiders in a Hearing World** (1980) comes to mind. There is undoubtedly a "boom" in this area—and more Deaf people writing books and theses, certainly an encouraging sign.[2]

You may wonder if hearing people can be part of Deaf culture. Indeed, they can. Parents and families of deaf children, friends, supporters, and advocates, can all be part of the Deaf community. Deaf culture is by no means restricted to deaf "members only."

Consider such educational giants of the past as Thomas Hopkins Gallaudet, Edward Miner Gallaudet, and Harvey P. Peet. All of them devoted their energies and considerable gifts to furthering the cause of Deaf education. Without them, our history (and the state of our culture) would have been immeasurably poorer.[3]

Hearing children of Deaf parents (like E.M. Gallaudet) often grow up with a strong affiliation to the Deaf community. Many of these individuals are native ASL users and bilingually proficient in ASL and English; they Sign so fluently as to be indistinguishable from Deaf people. Some choose careers as professional interpreters; others, another deaf-oriented profession such as teaching, social work, or advocacy. They straddle both Deaf and Hearing cultures. One notable example is the NTD performer, author, and ASL teacher, Lou Fant. Certain hearing educators, researchers, advocates, politicians, and "good neighbors" (like Sen. Tom Harkin of Iowa or Professors Harlan Lane, William Stokoe, and Ursula Bellugi) can become honorary members of the Deaf community, part of Deaf culture, even heroes.

1 Dr. Allen E. Sussman, Co-Director, Mental Health Counseling Program at Gallaudet University, made some timely remarks at a 1991 conference:

> For too long the field of deafness, including education, rehabilitation, psychology and mental health, has been preoccupied with what is wrong with deaf people rather than what is right with them. Authorities and experts in the field are experts in what's wrong with them, but their experience in what's right with them appears to be lacking. This pathological view is perpetuated by the same experts and authorities, many of whom are not able to communicate meaningfully with deaf children and adults.
>
> Moreover, the psychopathological perspective is rampantly manifest in the literature on deafness, especially in psychosocial aspects of deafness. There are several books, book chapters, and professional journal articles and almost all are pathologically oriented, dwelling on the problems and liabilities from language deficiency to behavior disorders. The focus is on the capital D's such as: Disability, Dysfunction, Deficiency and Deviance. Most "Psychology of Deafness" and related courses in graduate training programs are also pathologically oriented, depicting deaf children and adults in largely unfavorable light, further contributing to this distortion and imbalance. The emphasis, again, is on what they *cannot do* rather than on what they can do; the emphasis is on *liability* rather than *assets* which many deaf people possess in overwhelming abundance.

—Allen E. Sussman, Ph.D., "Characteristics of a well-adjusted Deaf Person, or: The Art of Being a Deaf Person," paper presented at the first National Conference on Childhood Deafness, Sioux Falls, South Dakota, April 1991, and reprinted in **DEAF LIFE**, July 1991.

2 Carol Padden and Tom Humphries, **Deaf in America: Voices from a Culture**. Cambridge, Massachusetts: Harvard University Press, 1988.

Paul C. Higgins, **Outsiders in a Hearing World: A Sociology of Deafness**. Beverly Hills: Sage Publications, 1980.

See also:

Jerome D. Schein, **At Home Among Strangers**. Washington, D.C.: Gallaudet University Press, 1989.

Sherman Wilcox, **American Deaf Culture: An Anthology**. Silver Spring, Md.: Linstok Press, 1989.

[3] Peet headed the New York School for the Deaf (Fanwood) from 1831 to 1866, transforming it into a first-rate institution. One of the great early leaders in Deaf education, he began his career in 1822 at the American School for the Deaf (Hartford).

Chapter 38

Should a hearing person write about Deaf Culture?

 ood question. If only insiders wrote about their own culture, the fields of sociology, anthropology, ethnology, and linguistics wouldn't exist! White scholars have written about Black culture, men about women's lives and literature, and non-Jews about Jewish history. Are their works without value because they were not "insiders"? Of course not. It may be brilliant, insightful, and eminently worthwhile. A researcher's objectivity and lack of preconceptions can be definite advantages. Yet an insider's view *is* important. To get a full picture, we want to balance the outsiders' views with what the insiders have to say.

Until fairly recently, everything that was written and published about Deaf culture was the work of "the Hearing." Should this analyzing of and "opinionating" about Deaf culture continue? It's not likely to stop. Is it good for us? Yes and no. Alexander Graham Bell used his meticulous research on the Deaf community *against* it. He and other oralists almost succeeded in wiping out Deaf culture. So powerful and influential was he that his notorious pamphlet, **Memoir Upon the Formation of a Deaf Variety of the Human Race**, is still being discussed! And ASL still has not made a complete comeback. It has not yet been fully restored to the classroom. (To a large extent, neither have Deaf teachers. There are still too few.)

On a brighter note, contemporary hearing scholars as

Harry Best,* William Stokoe, Ursula Bellugi, and Harlan Lane have certainly benefited the Deaf community and gained international respect for ASL and its culture. Hearing sociologists and linguists are now paying more attention to the Deaf community. Those who don't know ASL do field work with an interpreter. It's a booming field.

Some Deaf people feel suspicious of being made the subject of hearing scholars' studies, and understandably so. Sign language is the one thing that genuinely belongs to Deaf people, and it is the core of our identity. We have been robbed and cheated for nearly a century, and we don't want to lose it again. We do have the choice to cooperate or not in other people's research. We have the right to question the uses such research is put to.

But the best solution is for more Deaf people to master the complexities of written English, get advanced degrees, do scholarly studies on their own culture and community, publish them, and teach. This is happening. Much yet remains to be done. As the saying goes, the truth shall make us free.

* "Dr. Harry Best was a noted sociologist at the University of Kentucky. His **Deafness and the Deaf in the United States** (New York: Macmillan, 1943) was long considered *the definitive work* on the subject." —Dr. Robert F. Panara

Yours and Ours
(a few words to prospective researchers)

Traditionally, deaf people have been the subjects, the clients, the patients, the figures in statistics, the inferior class. Those who had the power—the theorists, scientist, researchers, educators, bureaucrats—were hearing. That is changing, and it's certainly a change for the better. More Deaf people are choosing to do scholarly studies of their own community. We feel that this is a healthy trend. But meanwhile, what about the majority—the Hearing majority? You will, of course, continue to be intrigued by the Deaf community, to study it, document it, compile statistics, and do field work and follow-up studies. That in itself is not bad. If it contributes to the sum of universal knowledge, we're all for it.

The root of all prejudice is the inability to accept human differences. Our major problems with the Hearing community can be traced to its refusal to accept our differences. If they don't recognize our language, for example, they won't have much respect for our need for accessible communication.

We don't ask that all hearing people learn sign language. We have no intention of forcing it on them. It's something that should be approached with enthusiasm and positive feelings, not out of fear of being slapped with a lawsuit under the ADA, nor a feeling of political/bureaucratic compulsion, nor because it's "trendy." We only ask that anyone who seeks to write about our history, our community, our language, make a genuine effort to understand why we feel the way we do, why we communicate as we do, why we have the problems we are currently entangled with, and where they came from.

If you look upon deafness merely as a lamentable condition—"one of the most desperate of human calamities," as Dr. Samuel Johnson described it—you may be moved to tearful pity at the thought that we cannot enjoy the pitter-patter of rain on the roof at night, the song of the lark, or the whispered words of love. With all due respect to these goodly things, to dwell on the lack or loss of them is to miss the whole point. We don't see ourselves as suffering sensory deprivation—that is, unless we sustain a sudden or progressive loss of hearing, in which case we have a whole life to set back into order. Many Deaf people do not mourn their lack of hearing; they see themselves as whole persons, not wounded ears. It may surprise you that a good number of Deaf people, when asked if they would choose to become hearing if they could, say no; they cannot imagine themselves any other way. We are deaf, and deaf is what we are. "Deaf" is a part of our rich and complex total identity as individuals. To us, being deaf is simply another way of being human. To someone who adheres to the medical-pathological view, deafness is a disability, a disorder, something negative. To us, it is simply a part of our personalities. Among ourselves, we don't make a big *shpiel* about it; it becomes subsumed in our everyday reality. It becomes invisible.

We *are* forcibly reminded of our deafness when we venture out into the Hearing world—when we tune into a cable-TV program that is not closed-captioned, when we are unable to find a pay telephone with a built-in TTY, when we find ourselves in a roomful of hearing people, none of whom can communicate with us. At times like this, we may find ourselves wishing that we could hear, if only to be free of the frustrations of having to cope endlessly with the Hearing world. Unfortunately, some hearing people, meeting us for the first time, never get beyond the fact of our deafness. It is a barrier, a wall.

Deaf people enjoy being different in the same sense that any ethnic minority enjoys being different from the majority. We enjoy and cherish ASL; we feel close kinship with our schoolmates; we have our jokes and fun, our pride. We have an identity. We have our disagreements, our squabbles, our ongoing philosophical feuds. As we have mentioned, some of it is very in-group stuff, not easily shared with outsiders. But that's true of any group.

We have much to teach society-at-large about things like cognition, language acquisition, neurolinguistics, thought patterns, and communication. And about oppression, prejudice, and the harvest that is reaped from years of low expectations.

Our concern here is attitude. If you *really* want to study the Deaf community, it's a good idea to learn Sign and become a part of our community in some way. Come as a student with an open mind, not as a judge. We welcome advocates and supporters, students and friends.

Chapter 39

"How did Alexander Graham Bell almost succeed in wiping out Deaf Culture?"

I have received the article titled "Should a hearing person write about Deaf Culture?" [See Chapter 38.] I have read several articles by your company & have learned a great deal about the Deaf Culture.

My question is this: in this particular article it mentioned Alexander Graham Bell almost succeeded in wiping out Deaf Culture. I would like to know how! I have obtained the article referred to & still can't see how that has set back the Deaf Culture. Perhaps you can point out to me what I am missing in that interpretation.

C. A., Tucson, Arizona

 ith the founding of the American School for the Deaf in Hartford in 1817, Deaf education in America began in earnest, and so did the Deaf Community. ASL was used to teach English in the classrooms; some of the best students stayed on after graduation and became teachers; and Hartford-trained teachers and administrators helped set up other schools for the deaf across the country. Educated deaf people entered a variety of professions. The "silent press" began publishing. Deaf clubs were founded. There was considerable interest in founding a college for deaf people.

After a brief "golden age" (1830s-1860s), ASL-based Deaf education came under attack from Alexander Graham Bell and other wealthy and powerful oralists. The oral movement in the States had emerged during the 1860s, and the Milan Congress of 1880 gave it added impetus. Bell, who founded the American Association to Promote the Teaching of Speech to the Deaf (now called the Alexander Graham Bell Association for the Deaf) was the leading oral advocate.

Bell was a brilliant inventor and indefatigable social theorist—famous, wealthy, and enormously influential. Although he was a skillful Signer and acknowledged the beauty of sign language, he believed that speech was of supreme importance, and that deaf people should assimilate into hearing society. According to Gallaudet University historians John Van Cleve and Barry Crouch, "Bell believed that deafness was a terrible curse . . . a pathological aberration [that] perpetuated negative genetic traits . . . that deaf persons weakened the society in which they lived."* After studying records of several schools for the deaf, he compiled his notorious paper, **Memoir Upon the Formation of a Deaf Variety of the Human Race** (1883). He desired to put a stop to the "alarming" growth of Deaf culture and prevent deaf children from being born. Accordingly, he proposed legislation against "the intermarriage of congenital deaf-mutes." Since he doubted this would work, he suggested three "preventive measures": eliminating residential schools, forbidding the use of sign language in the education of deaf pupils, and prohibiting deaf adults from being teachers of deaf children. His proposals almost succeeded.

The oralists wielded considerable political and educational influence. Inexorably, the tide turned against Signing residential schools, and the Deaf community found itself outnumbered and outmaneuvered, as well as out-moneyed. The efforts of Bell and his colleagues led to the spread of oral day schools. And by the turn of the century, the majority of residential schools in the United States had switched to the oral method—sometimes forcibly. By 1919, the peak of the oralist "wave," 80% of residential schools had "gone oral." Deaf teachers had been forced out of the profession. Sign language was prohibited in classes. If students were caught Signing, they were punished. Of course, they continued to Sign with each other, but had to do it covertly—in the dorms at night, or in the toilets. All of which had profoundly negative effects on their self-esteem.

Bell wasn't directly responsible for this oppression, but as an advocate, he paved the way. He helped empower the oral movement, funded it, and gave it credibility. His ideas, though, have not stood the test of time. Although residential schools are yet again under attack, ASL is alive and well, its artistry thriving. We wonder what Bell would have said about the numbers of hearing high-school and college students taking ASL as a foreign language! The National Theatre of the Deaf recently celebrated its silver anniversary. We are emerging from the "dark age" of the past century—but slowly.

Even Clarke School, that bastion of oralism, finally recognized the futility of suppressing sign language; it has dropped its old policy of penalizing students who were caught signing. Although signing is still not allowed in class, students can sign freely outside of class without fear of punishment. In signing residential schools, there is a definite trend towards the Bilingual-Bicultural model, which is in many ways a throwback to the Hartford model: using ASL to teach English.

*John Vickrey Van Cleve and Barry A. Crouch, **A Place of their Own: Creating the Deaf Community in America**, p. 145. See also Richard Winefield, **Never the Twain Shall Meet: The Communications Debate**.

Chapter 40

At my daughter's wedding, I saw my nephew dance for the first time, and I was surprised to see him dancing so beautifully. How could he do that if he's deaf? My sister tried to explain how that could work. I still don't understand. Can all deaf people dance like him?

e personally enjoy seeing people doing what others imagine unthinkable—wrecking stereotypical notions of what's normal "handicapped" behavior. But the fact is that deaf people are very much individuals, and exactly like hearing people in that respect. And while some hearing people are terrific dancers and some are incredible klutzes, the same applies to deaf people. Some are just so physically *free*, so beautifully coordinated, so creative with movement, that they've made professional or quasi-professional careers out of dance, while others equally deaf are stiff and awkward—hippopotami on skateboards. Since deafness can affect the sense of balance whose center is in the inner ear, many deaf people must struggle especially hard to achieve coordination and grace—and sometimes this makes them better, more motivated dancers!*

We can learn to dance very well without being able to

hear the music. What's required is a sharp eye, alertness, sensitivity to rhythm, and coordination—the same skills any good dancer develops. Dance classes set up for deaf students use visual cues, amplified music (with a vigorous bass section), and a lot of percussion—like tambour drums—that sends very strong vibrations through the air and can be felt in one's bones (particularly the breastbone). On stage, without the help of the drum, they can keep mental count.

That deaf dancers "feel the vibrations through the floor" is something of a misconception. Since their feet are not in contact with the floor at all times, it's more accurate to say deaf dancers feel vibrations of the music through their bodies. They learn to keep a sharp eye-corner on what's happening, as well as developing and refining their intuitive, "internalized" sense of rhythm. Your nephew was keenly alert to what was going on and used his own everyday skills to keep perfect pace with the others.

Anyone who says that deaf people can't dance is a dolt. And anyone who says that *all* deaf people *are* good dancers is a bigger dolt.

---

*As an example of what a deaf dancer can achieve, we can look at the remarkable career of Frances Woods (b. 1907). Woods (real name: Esther Thomas) was born totally deaf, yet became a professional dancer in 1926. She and her hearing husband, Billy Bray (real name: Anthony Caliguire), formed a team, dancing in hotels and taverns during the Depression, then in vaudeville (live routines) the R.K.O. chain of theaters. Their routines included acrobatics, mime, and a variety of elements from popular dances of the day. Woods designed and made all her own costumes. Robert L. Ripley (of "Believe It Or Not!" fame), called them the Wonder Dancers. Woods and Bray performed throughout the 1930s, 1940s, and 1950s, in many famous nightclubs and hotels, accompanied by some of the great bands, in the States and Europe. They even played in London's famed Palladium. Even after retirement, they were still dancing together.

See Robert F. Panara's entries on Woods and "Dance" (Performing Arts) in the **Gallaudet Encyclopedia of Deaf People and Deafness**, and his collection of biographies (with John Panara), **Great Deaf Americans** (Silver Spring, Md.: T.J. Publishers, 1983).

Chapter 11

Are Deaf people visually sharper than Hearing people?

he #1 favorite misconception about disabled people seems to be that when you've lost use of one sense, the other senses magically become stronger. There's no real magic here, just practicality. A blind person develops acute skill in using the remaining senses—touch, smell, hearing, a sensitivity to changes in the air—to live a full life. They don't really develop some kind of preternatural sonar. They use the capabilities everyone has. Likewise, Deaf people learn to rely on visual cues. This doesn't make them visually smarter or eagle-eyed. They simply become more alert about taking in and processing visual messages. Paying close attention and noticing easily overlooked details is a survival skill. And not all deaf people are good at it, either.

If all deaf people were visually gifted, they'd all be artists and terrific drivers. Of course, this isn't so. While it's true that many deaf students choose design-oriented careers, many have no aptitude whatsoever. Although statistically, deaf people tend to be better drivers than hearing ones, some deaf drivers can be just as sloppy and careless as any hearing counterpart. We know color-blind and artistically untalented deaf people; we know bad drivers and careful ones.

Nor do you have to be deaf to acquire skill in ASL, which is a visually-based language (as English is an aurally-based—spoken—one). Hearing children of Deaf parents who grow up using ASL every day naturally develop a high degree of skill, while deaf people who learn to sign later in life often lack that facility. It's not a question of innate genius but exposure and practice.

Deaf people use their eyes as hearing people use their ears. While hearing people tend to rely more on their hearing than vision, deaf people rely exclusively on their eyes. Alert Deaf signers tend to take better notice of the persons they're communicating with—the nuances of expression, the momentary glances, the subtle changes in posture that indicate a change in mood or a dwindling of attention.

It should be noted that there are a number of visual impairments that are genetically linked to deafness. Usher's syndrome type 2 is perhaps the best-known of these. It is a fairly rare recessive genetic condition. To transmit Usher's, both parents (who will have normal hearing) must carry a similar abnormal gene. The affected person is born profoundly deaf, and gradually loses sight, suffering night blindness during early adolescence, a progressive narrowing of the field of vision ("tunnel vision"), becoming completely blind. Usher's syndrome is a form of *retinitis pigmentosa*—abnormal deposits of pigment causing damage to the retina (the exceptionally delicate light-sensitive portion of the eye), and the loss of peripheral vision. About half of all deaf-blind people have Usher's syndrome, as do some 3% to 6% of all congenitally deaf children. There is no treatment, nor can it be identified before birth. Many of us know several people who have Usher's syndrome.

Two much less common conditions that also affect both hearing and vision are Cogan's syndrome and Alport's disease. Cogan's syndrome is an inflammation of the cornea which can also damage the delicate organs of the inner ear—the *organ of Corti* and *cochlear nerve cells*—resulting in vertigo, tinnitus, and sensorineural hearing loss ("nerve-deafness"). This can be treated with steroid drugs. Alport's disease, more common in men than women, involves kidney inflammation in childhood, sensorineural hearing loss in early adulthood, and eye problems later in life.

Some deaf people (whom we know personally) are color-blind; some have dyslexia.

Therefore, it is ridiculous to generalize about the "supersensitive" visual skills of *all* deaf people. Vision problems and progressive blindness are a fact of life for many deaf people. A number of deaf people may not even be aware that they *have* a vision problem, either. This is due to the old lack of communication between medical personnel and deaf children. NTID, for example, requires *all* incoming freshmen to have their eyes tested. It's not unknown for the medical staff to detect and diagnose conditions that eluded previous examiners—if nobody ever bothered to explain things clearly to the deaf person, or to ask the right questions in an easily understandable way, neither the doctors nor the patient gets the full picture.

The only thing that can accurately be said of *all* deaf people as a whole is that since they can't hear, they rely on sight, lights, vibration, and other tactile means to function normally.

Chapter 42

What difficulties do deaf people have when driving an automobile? Why is their insurance higher than a hearing person's? And do deaf people take the same test as hearing people?

eaf people have been driving automobiles since the first ones rolled out at the turn of the century. According to **Deaf Heritage**, during the 1920s (a time of steadily increasing automobile accidents and fatalities), at least four states refused to license deaf drivers, and other states considered doing likewise. Deaf drivers ultimately won the right to drive in all states. As their good driving records became more widely known, hostility against them decreased.

Charging deaf people more for insurance is an old problem. The National Fraternal Society of the Deaf (FRAT) was founded in 1898 as a response to discriminatory life-insurance practices. (Deaf drivers aren't *necessarily* charged more because they're deaf. We suggest you check with hearing friends who share your insurance company, compare their rates, and see if there really is a difference. There are many factors involved in these rates, such as whether the car is new, old, or a Rolls-Royce.)

Currently, the major problem seems to be the discrimination deaf drivers face when trying to purchase a new car. Some dealers still refuse to allow them to test-drive a new car, supposedly because they're "risky." The Americans with Disabilities Act, which went into effect January 26, 1992, prohibits discrimination on the basis of disability. New-car dealers are required to eliminate architectural and communication barriers, provide auxiliary aids as needed, and ensure equal access to any transportation service provided to other customers. But it remains to be seen exactly what sort of impact the ADA will have here. Some new-car dealers are aware of the law; others aren't, but don't anticipate any particular problems, as they welcome all customers. We anticipate a number of lawsuits by deaf and disabled consumers against auto dealers who are not complying with the law.

Are the fears of the jittery dealers founded? Statistics show that deaf drivers are just as good as hearing drivers, and, on the whole, a better safety risk. (*Now* can we have the keys?)

Although some hearing folks are surprised to learn that deaf people can drive, the fact is, driving is an almost completely visual activity for anyone. (How many drivers watch the road with their ears, anyway?) Hearing drivers routinely close their windows when the air-conditioning is on, effectively masking out auditory clues. CD players, cassette decks, radios, and cellular phones also mask outside noises. Trucks are much noisier than cars, and some truck drivers wear protective earplugs.

Under such circumstances, a hearing driver is in much the same situation as a deaf driver. But a deaf driver may have an advantage. Deaf persons "are already highly skilled in compensating for their hearing loss at all times by increased visual alertness."* Lacking auditory distractions, they tend to concentrate better. Studies have corroborated this. A 1968 study of every deaf driver in the Washington, D.C. area over a 3-year period "produced evidence that the deaf drivers had less than one-third as many accidents and only one-half as many traffic tickets as non-deaf drivers."

Deaf drivers can carry on animated conversations in Sign with other passengers. Although this involves momentarily glancing away from the road, it's quite safe. Most Deaf passengers will share the responsibility of keeping watch with the driver and are quick to alert him or her; everybody looks after each other.

Licensing tests vary from state to state, but we've never heard of any deaf person being turned down for a license solely because they're deaf. They take the same tests a hearing driver does. New York State driver's licenses, for example, list one or more pertinent restrictions: if a driver wears a hearing aid while driving, that will be noted, and all deaf drivers are required to have three full-view mirrors.

*Particular thanks to NICD and FRAT for the information utilized here. Quotes are taken from various articles excerpted by FRAT.

Chapter 43

Don't Deaf people have to wear dark colors?

rofessional interpreters, most of whom are hearing, do have a dress code for their job. To ensure that their signing remains as visible as possible, they usually wear solid colors. These don't have to be dark, just as long as they provide an unobtrusive background to their signing. Interpreters will try to avoid wearing anything that could render their Signing less distinct, or, heaven forbid, cause visual annoyance to the Deaf "signee."

Some college interpreters actually don a baggy black smock while on duty. Some Deaf people find this practice distasteful, as it promotes an unattractive image of interpreters. We prefer to see interpreters wearing nice professional-looking outfits—or even casual shirts, sweaters, jerseys, or dresses. They DON'T have to be black; they can be dark blue, navy, deep purple, gray—any quiet, unobtrusive color which makes a good foil to the play of the hands and face.

Red and white are out. Flesh colors—peach, blush, some shades of tan and brown—are definitely out. So are hot (neon) colors, bold stripes, and loud, splashy patterns, which can give the Deaf "signee" a headache. Some male interpreters wear ties; many don't, to avoid too much "busyness" in the signing space of the upper torso. Many interpreters wear gold jewelry, including rings; jewelry isn't necessarily a distraction. Wristwatches are okay.

Theatrical and artistic interpreters, whose signing has

to be visible across the distance of a theater hall or auditorium, often wear dark solids. Black is especially popular, especially for "shadow" interpreters, who are onstage right there with the costumed performers— clearly visible but as visually unobtrusive as possible. Deaf performers (i.e., ASL poets) will often choose similar dark solids. But there are no real hard-and fast rules here, just the requisite of visibility. We've seen very colorfully-costumed National Theatre of the Deaf productions.

NTD is very careful about the design of its costumes. All costumes for Deaf theatre must take into account the readability of the signing (hands and face), and the lighting. Costumes have to provide a good background for the signing—not detract from or interfere with it. Proper lighting eliminates dark shadows across the upper torso, which would also interfere with the clarity of the signing. Clarity and visibility are the guiding principles of all Deaf-oriented theatre and TV productions.

For TV productions, by the way, different rules apply for different audiences. In a normal "Hearing" TV production, you can have a tightly-cropped close-up of the face. But with a Signed/ASL production, you can't. The shot has to include not only the face but the signing space as well—which includes the whole upper half of the body. (See Chapter 10). This limits the artistic flexibility of the camera. Close-up shots, so dear to filmmakers and TV, must be scrupulously avoided.

For Deaf people in everyday, off-the-job life, there are no rules and no restrictions. They wear what they like. If brightly-striped rugby shirts and Hawaiian prints are popular with young hearing people, they're popular with young Deaf people too. On a normal conversational basis, neons, polka dots, jungle prints, picture T-shirts, even garish tie-dyes, don't present a real problem. Some especially strident shirt-patterns or colors do make it difficult to see someone's Signing across a distance. But ski masks, sunglasses, and hats that obscure the eyes, as well as thick, unruly beards and sweeping mustaches, may very well interfere with close-range communication. Sunglasses, hats, and masks, at least, are easily slipped off!

By the way, skilled Signers can carry on conversations while wearing mittens . . . but that's another story.

Chapter 44

"Do deaf people show a slight difference in their facial anatomy?"

I have often noticed a slight (but in no way unattractive) anatomical difference on many deaf, Deaf, and hard-of-hearing people. The upper lip is thinner or slightly turned up, and there are sometimes slight variations of the nostrils.

In my narrow "heary" range of experience, it seems to be more common among the hard-of-hearing than the Deaf. Is this caused by the medical problems that cause hearing loss or is it caused by the way the face is strained while trying to vocalize or hear other people? My Daughter, who experienced severe trauma in one ear as a 5-year-old, has developed this trait. Again, I do not find this to be unattractive. In my totally unbiased opinion, I have a very beautiful daughter.

—a reader in Albuquerque, New Mexico

his is a fascinating question (actually, there are several psycho-socio-anthropological questions here), because it touches on some very subtle aspects of hearing loss: the possible differences between the way deaf and hearing people *look*.

Deafness has been called "the invisible handicap," and not without reason. It has long been argued that deaf people are not immediately recognizable as "deaf"— *unless* they wear hearing aids or other visible devices, clothing proclaiming their status as students of deaf institutions, "ILY" or "Deaf Culture" pins, or other identifiers. And, of course, unless they're seen Signing in public.

This reader asks about the upper lip, and the nostrils. From our experience (and we've met and interacted with hundreds upon hundreds of other Deaf, deaf, and hard-of-hearing people), we've found no evidence that they have thinner or more upturned upper lips than hearing people do. Or that their nostrils are unequal. A deaf or deafened person can certainly have a medical condition that affects the facial muscles, but we don't know any instances of deafness *itself* causing this kind of facial change. We'd call it deafness *in combination with* some other condition. "Medical problems that cause hearing loss" usually leave no telltale signs on the face. Otherwise, why do so many deaf children get misdiagnosed? It's just not visible.

We do note, however, that deaf people (on the whole) use their facial muscles differently from hearing people. In ASL, the entire face is used as a grammatical marker. The eyebrows, for example, are used to indicate questions, and the way the eyebrows are raised or knit and the head tilted specifies what kind of question it is. All this is subtle and momentary. Native ASL users employ a fleeting nostril-twitch to indicate "Yes, I agree with you." Like the eyebrows, the nose is used as a unit of communication, so the nostrils may be momentarily dilated and "up-twitched," singly, during the conversational give-and-take. In contrast, when hearing people talk to each other, the nostrils are *supposed* to be relaxed. Twitchy nostrils are a seen as a symptom of stress or facial tic.

Facial expressions depend on the mode of communication as well as the mood of the communicator. Hard-of-hearing people, who have a hearing loss but struggle to function normally within hearing parameters, might well strain to attend, listen, and enunciate clearly; the tension would certainly be perceptible in their faces. ASL users have particularly intense-looking facial expressions because, as we've just noted, the face is employed grammatically. Uneducated hearing onlookers who happen to observe a real ASL conversation will sometimes say that the conversationalists "look angry at each other," even when it's a perfectly friendly chat.

Our facial muscles are extraordinarily flexible. We've all seen actors who so literally identify with their characters that they assume the habitual expressions of those characters—even "between takes."* The same goes for deaf and hard-of-hearing people: the demands of communication impose their visible signs on the expressions of the face. But if a deaf or hard-of-hearing person's face is in repose (i.e., idly waiting for a bus, reading, watching TV, or gazing into a computer screen), we don't think there are *any* distinguishing characteristics between a deaf face and a hearing one.

*We recall reading an article in a popular magazine so years ago focusing on the sometimes-astonishing resemblance between wives and husbands. After associating intimately with each other for years, their facial expressions tend to reflect each other's; certain expressive "configurations" become habitual.

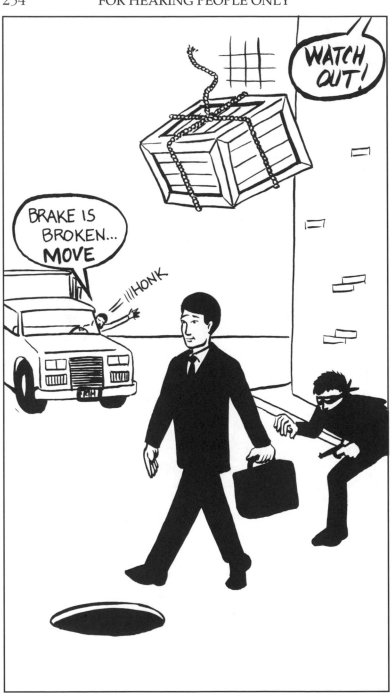

Chapter 45

Aren't deaf people more prone to accidents?

n the last century it was commonly, and mistakenly, believed that deaf people had shorter-than-average lifespans. Insurance companies considered them high risks—more accident-prone than hearing people—and accordingly charged them more.

It is true that deaf persons are more vulnerable in *some* circumstances. Every so often, you read a newspaper item about a deaf man or woman who was shot to death in a mugging or robbery. Too often, the criminal orders the victim to do something—"Don't move!" or "Lie down!"—without realizing that the deaf person can't hear the command. Especially from behind. When the deaf victim fails to comply, s/he gets killed, and another tragic crime story ends up in the newspapers. The effect of such stories, unfortunately, is to reinforce the stereotype of deaf people being helpless, pathetic, and easily victimized.

Sometimes it *can* make a difference if a victim is able to inform the assailants that s/he is deaf. In **I Didn't Hear the Dragon Roar**, Frances M. "Peggy" Parsons tells of how she narrowly escaped being knifed to death in Mozambique. Having disregarded a warning not to walk alone in the dark, she went downtown, took a "wrong exit" from a department store, and was attacked in a narrow alley by "three surly young men with tribal scars across their faces." One brandished a knife. She struggled to get one hand free and gestured that she was deaf. The man with the knife signed, "You deaf? Me have deaf sister." He ordered his accomplices to release her, helped her to her feet, returned her purse, asked her what she was doing in Mozambique, and kissed her hand in parting, saying, "You saint. No walk alone!"*

As for fires: deaf people, particularly poor children and the elderly who live in unsafe buildings without proper smoke-alarm hookups, are indeed vulnerable. Smoke alarms are available with flashing "strobe" signals that are virtually impossible to "miss," even if you're asleep. Some single persons and families have a hearing-ear dog—a dependable mongrel or pedigree working-breed who is specially trained to respond to noises and alert its owners. (A good dog is worth its weight in gold. How many lives—whether deaf or hearing—have been saved by "ordinary" family pooches?!)

In some ways, deaf people may have definite advantages over their hearing counterparts—e.g., job safety. Alert deaf people keep their eyes open and their reflexes sharp. However, it must be said that not all deaf people *are* alert. Some are careless, lethargic, and clumsy. These become the "accident-prone" folks of the stereotype.

Some forms of deafness also affect the center of balance in the inner ear, which entails both impaired hearing *and* balance. Such people have difficulty walking in the dark, and need light to see.

The center of balance is located in the inner ear, in the fluid-filled *semicircular canals* and *labyrinth* attached to the cochlea, which controls hearing. Inflammation of inner-ear tissue, degeneration of nerve or auditory "hair" cells, or abnormal buildup of fluid (perilymph), will accordingly affect a person's sense of balance.

Deaf people with poor balance who cope well in daylight or where there is good illumination at night, can get easily disoriented in darkness (e.g., during a blackout), where there is a lack of visual cues to guide them, and will often bump into things, stumble, fall, and get hurt.

Ménière's disease is one such condition that may affect both hearing and balance—a devastating combination. A person who has Ménière's experiences irregular attacks of dizziness, vertigo (a feeling of moving, whirling and rotating in space), nausea, and tinnitus (annoying, obtrusive noises in the inner ear). Such people, needless to say, may experience an attack at any time.

Deaf people are not more prone to accidents just *because* they're deaf. A multiplicity of factors is involved.

*Frances M. Parsons, **I Didn't Hear the Dragon Roar** (1988), xii.

Chapter 46

Why do so many Deaf people work in printing, post-office, or factory jobs?

or many years, printing was considered the ideal job for a deaf man. Most residential schools for the deaf had their own print shops and published Deaf newsletters, newspapers, and journals—the legendary "Little Papers." Printing paid well, even during the Depression. And it offered prestige. Printers were "the elite." Many deaf men became skilled Linotypists. (Presumably, deaf Linotypists could better concentrate on their work without being bothered by the extremely noisy machines.) But with the revolution in cold type and desktop publishing, and the phasing-out of Linotype machines, printing has ceased to be the "natural" choice. Nonetheless, it's still a popular one.

The second most common traditional vocation for deaf boys—shoemaking—is history now.*

For deaf girls, very few of whom entered the printing field (not that they were encouraged!), dressmaking/ seamstressing was considered the ideal ticket to financial independence in the event they couldn't snag a husband. In the days before off-the-rack clothing offered a wide variety of sizes, it was, no doubt, an indispensable skill.

Teaching the deaf was a respected profession for Deaf adults—that is, until the "victory" of oralism a century ago. As a result of the schools' mass switch to the oral method, Deaf people were gradually forced out of the profession. Even today, the overwhelming majority of teachers of the deaf are hearing.

Many deaf people still work in blue-collar trades. They tend to seek jobs known to be "open to the deaf." The Post Office is the nation's largest single employer of deaf people. Factories (at least until the latest recession) always needed workers. Deaf people like to work with other deaf people. And there is peer pressure to conform. Certain jobs are "socially acceptable." Others aren't. Members of the local Deaf community may look askance at a deaf person who "steps out of line."

As a result of many factors, relatively few deaf people have ventured into non-traditional ("white-collar") careers. Progress has been notably irregular. The doors of opportunity, which were not exactly flung wide, are slowly opening. Slowly. Deaf children are still subjected to low expectations—"A pilot? Don't be silly. Deaf people can't be pilots!" "You can't be a TV producer—you're deaf!" As young adults, they face discrimination, blatant and subtle. By this time, many have developed a self-image problem. How many employers refuse to hire a third Deaf person because of bad experiences with the first two? Even very motivated, enthusiastic Deaf people may be badly educated and ill-prepared. And in today's competitive job market, "fighting spirit" alone isn't quite enough. Support, networking, and role models are still in short supply. And many Deaf people seem quite content with the "old ways." Fewer risks mean less frustration, pain, and disappointment.

About 10 years ago, a hearing oralist educator expressed the common view that the world wasn't likely to accommodate to deaf people by learning *their* language; deaf people have to accommodate to the hearing world. He pointed out that his daughter, who was deaf, had a good job at a major corporation, and that she'd never have been able to get that job if she couldn't talk. Fortunately, this arrogant attitude isn't true anymore. More employers are willing to take a risk by hiring a deaf worker. Good speech is no longer seen as the main criterion of a deaf person's success in the Hearing world. Talent is.

Despite a sluggish national economy, layoffs, closedowns, and rising unemployment (the disturbing stuff we read about and see on the news), we'd have to say that the Deaf job outlook is reasonably bright. Computer/imaging technologies and other high-tech fields are expanding the opportunities for deaf people; more and more students are entering them. Computer technologies have helped create a wider job market for deaf people. The Americans with Disabilities Act will, we believe, encourage big companies to hire more deaf people. The Deaf community contains a pool of talent that has scarcely begun to be tapped.

*For a biography of one such Deaf man, see Harvey Barash and Eva Barash Dicker, **Our Father Abe: The Story of a Deaf Shoe Repairman** (1991).

▲ ▲ ▲

NTID and the "Techie" Option

The idea of higher education for deaf people became a reality in 1864, when President Lincoln signed the charter for what is now Gallaudet University. Gallaudet was, and still is, the only 4-year liberal-arts college in the world for deaf people.

While many hearing people know about Gallaudet (which seems to capture the lion's share of publicity),

262 FOR HEARING PEOPLE ONLY

not too many are aware of the existence of the National Technical Institute for the Deaf (NTID), which is one of 8 colleges of Rochester Institute of Technology. NTID was founded specifically to address the problem of deaf people's under-employment in skilled technical trades. P.L. 89-36, the law creating NTID, was signed by President Lyndon B. Johnson in 1965, and just in the nick of time, too. A nationwide rubella (German measles) epidemic during the mid-1960s resulted in an unusually large number of deaf and multiply-handicapped babies. By the time these children of the "rubella bulge" were ready to enter college in the summer of 1984, NTID was prepared for them. (The first students were admitted in 1968.) While Gallaudet attracts more students from a traditional Deaf-cultural residential-school milieu, NTID's appeal is more eclectic; its deaf population comes from from a wide range of backgrounds (i.e., more mainstreaming). Like Gallaudet, NTID now accepts Canadian and foreign students. The average deaf student population during the academic year is around 1,000.

Rochester, New York, is universally known as the home of Kodak. It's also the original home base of Bausch & Lomb (the giant optical company), IBM, and Xerox, which still maintain a presence there. NTID's host institution, RIT, maintains close ties with corporations like these. Largely because of NTID, Rochester also boasts the largest per-capita deaf population of any city in the U.S.

NTID students have a wide array of majors to choose from in four schools (Business, Engineering, Science, and Visual Communication). Many of the careers are in non-traditional, "bankable" fields, and NTID boasts that 95% of its graduates find appropriate employment. Majors include applied computer technology, applied accounting, electromechanical technology, architectural technology, civil technology, optical finishing technology, medical record technology, applied art, applied photography, media production technology, and printing production technology. NTID students can also cross-register into other RIT colleges, taking advantages of the available support services (interpreters, tutors, and notetakers).

No institution is perfect, but it can justly be said that NTID has opened up many new careers for deaf students and has, in its own way, helped eliminate stereotyping and negative beliefs. Students are reminded by their teachers and career counselors that upon graduation they may conceivably become the first deaf persons hired by their companies, and that their employers may well judge all deaf people by their behavior. It's a burden, yes, but also an opportunity to break new ground—and to excel.

Chapter 47

At the airport, I was approached by a Deaf person selling manual-alphabet cards. Should I buy one?

NO! NO!

any people in the Deaf community know someone who sells "ABC" cards for a living. That certainly doesn't stop us from feeling angry and resentful about it.

A peddler appears to be uneducated, unskilled, and unemployable, a pitiful victim of society. In truth, some of these peddlers are not uneducated, nor unskilled, nor unemployable. They're clever. By preying on the gullibility of hearing people, a successful peddler can earn $200—or more—a day! Card-peddlers like to frequent heavily trafficked places like airports, where a continuous stream of foreigners, newly arrived in the States, are getting their first glimpse of American society—and the first deaf person they meet is, for all practical purposes, a beggar. Small wonder that Deaf people, the majority of whom are hard-working taxpayers, bitterly resent the stereotype that these peddlers perpetuate.[1]

Deaf people have invested considerable time, energy, and passion into educating the Hearing public and attempting to undo the cumulative damage of centuries of negative, demeaning, and offensive images of the Deaf. It's an ongoing process. Along comes a peddler with a stack of cards, each one stating: "I AM A DEAF-MUTE." Is this how we want hearing people to think of us? In their own humble way, such individuals threaten to undermine all that Deaf people have labored to achieve, and all for the sake of monetary gain (their own or the head honcho who collects kickbacks). Who knows how many thousands of hearing folks without any prior knowledge of deafness have encountered these peddlers? Ambassadors of Deaf culture, indeed! Imagine the fear that strikes the heart of a mother or father whose child has just been diagnosed as deaf and who recalls encountering a peddler: Is my daughter or son going to become one of *them*?

There is a difference between voluntarily buying a trinket from a peddler at a sidewalk table or cart, and being psychologically pressured into "paying any price you wish" for a fuzzy ABC chart by someone who comes up to you in a shop or café. At least the stereotypical blind man selling pencils for 5¢ apiece at the street corner is offering something useful for the money.[2] We've noticed that none of these kind-hearted folks who bought ABC cards ever bothered to use them. (If they did, we'd have a legion of hearing people who could fingerspell!) ABC cards aren't a legitimate product like pencils or pot-holders. They're a gimmick. Selling them is a psychological con game. Hearing people who really want to learn the manual alphabet and to communicate with Deaf people shouldn't have to pay through the nose for it.[3]

In buying an ABC card, hearing people feel they're doing a good turn by helping a less fortunate person. One peddler's solicitation card (attached to a keychain) reads: "$1.00 contribution will be appreciated," implying that their money is going towards a non-profit cause. It isn't. The money they give peddlers is money that could be, but isn't, used for a really positive cause— buying a ticket to the National Theatre of the Deaf, a hand-crafted item made by an NTID student, a box of holiday cards designed by students from the nearest school for the deaf.

Just in case you need another reason not to shell out, we'd like to note that a good number of these "deaf" peddlers aren't even deaf. They're hearing persons faking deafness.

There's one thing that these peddlers can't seem to handle. When approaching a potential "soft touch" who asks them sternly in fluent ASL, "Why are you doing this?", the only thing they can do is mutter "Oh, sorry!" and make a quick escape.

Not all members of the Deaf community despise peddlers. Some feel that card-peddling should be tolerated, as it's part of our culture. It may not be the most prestigious way to make a living, they feel, but peddlers shouldn't be vilified. They are certainly accepted in the Deaf-club milieu. Some Deaf people resent them for "giving deaf people a bad name." But others admire them for wreaking revenge on the "Hearies" who exploit Deaf people. The bosses who operate peddling rings may exploit other Deaf people, but the peddlers themselves target hearing strangers exclusively. In other words: 'You cheat ours, so we're gonna cheat yours.' Unfortunately for this logic, the *real* exploiters and oppressors aren't the ones who get defrauded by the peddlers.

[1]See **Deaf Heritage,** pp. 255-259, for a historical survey of peddling that includes the poignant "Profile of a Deaf Peddler." There was an upsurge in deaf peddlers after World War II, as deaf factory workers were replaced *en masse* by returning war veterans. Major Deaf organizations tried to combat the peddling "epidemic" as forcefully they could.

[2]Peddlers don't necessarily limit themselves to ABC cards. They

can push small items like Band-Aids, combs, or keychains—all in return for a "suggested contribution" which is much more than the items are worth. The cute little keychain we saw, for example, was selling for a "suggested contribution" of $1.00. Not a bad profit for an item which cost the peddler perhaps 10¢.

[3]For example, NTID publishes an attractive brochure, "Let's Communicate: Basic Signs & Tips for Communicating with Deaf People," which contains clear illustrations of the manual alphabet, the numbers 1-10, and an assortment of basic signs. It's free for the asking.

Deaf Awareness: 5-Minute Quiz

Chapters 35—47

Answers are on the bottom of the page, upside down.

True or False:

1. Many ancient cultures considered deafness a curse; deaf people were treated as outcasts. In ancient Greece, a baby discovered to be deaf would have been unlikely to survive infancy.

2. There have been very, few sociological studies of the Deaf community, and certainly none by deaf people themselves.

3. Alexander Graham Bell, who wanted to wipe out deafness, disband the Deaf community, and assimilate all deaf people into the hearing world, was a skilled Signer who acknowledged the beauty of sign language.

4. Deaf people can make superb dancers, even without being able to hear the music.

5. Some "deaf" peddlers selling manual-alphabet cards aren't even deaf; they're faking it.

Answers:
1. True; 2. False; 3. True; 4. True; 5. True.

Chapter 48

I've noticed that successful deaf persons are always put down by other deaf people, by means of lack of support and gossip—back-stabbing, name-calling, nasty rumors. Can't deaf people appreciate successful achievers who benefit their community?

 he operative word here is "jealousy." Deaf culture embodies a "closed group"—small in numbers, linguistically unique, and mindful of their differences. Deaf people have traditionally tended to band together; thus the Deaf club, which has proven not just a vital social institution and positive means of sharing information and experiences and garnering support ("networking"), but less admirably, a hotbed of gossip, destructive rumor-mongering, and character assassination. Despite recent incursions from home-centered TV's and VCR's, the Deaf club is still a mainstay of the Deaf community. So is gossip.

Oppressed in blatant and subtle ways from a very early age, Deaf people have traditionally reacted by huddling into something like solidarity: "Let's endure this together; are we all here?" This group loyalty has in turn fostered a rigid conformist mentality. If I'm oppressed by the Hearing culture, and you're oppressed, we can help each other out, but if you do something to rock the boat or break loose from the group, even if it will ultimately benefit me, you've disrupted the order of things and behaved disloyally to your Deaf culture. I feel threatened by your success, and I'm jealous.

The situation is analogous to that of Black students in inner-city high schools who are serious about their schoolwork and trying to excel in academics—the kind of young I-really-want-to-go-to-college achievers everybody wants to encourage. Everybody? What kind of peer pressure are *they* experiencing? How much support do they get from the others? Not long ago, we saw a **World News Tonight** segment on the plight of these students, who complained about being verbally and physically harassed—even beaten up—by other Black students because they were seen as "nerds" or "trying to act white." They were under tremendous pressure to be part of the "gang," and when they refused, the gangies vented their wrath on them. It sounded eerily familiar.

Many Deaf people don't understand what "dreams" and "ambitions" are. They are schooled in lowered expectations almost from the start. (That is undoubtedly one reason why some parents of deaf children prefer the idea of mainstreaming, and not without reason—many residential schools for the deaf don't offer the same quality of academic challenge as public schools.) They have been conditioned to take the least challenging path: seek out a factory job, buy a house and car, and settle down, "just like everyone else." That's what's acceptable. Those who cherish a different dream—taking risks, moving into non-traditional ("Hearing") professions, rejecting the club mentality—may find themselves becoming targets for the most vicious imaginable brand of gossip.

But what starts as a "cultural" issue shades into a

moral one. Gossip says plenty—about the jealousy, bitterness, and weak characters of those who spread it. Well-adjusted, happy, mature individuals do not feel the need to project their own inadequacies onto others.

Chapter 49

I'm a student in a sign-language class. I've noticed that my deaf teacher uses the term "hearing" to describe me. I find it very strange that deaf people do that. Why do deaf people use the terms "hearing" and "hearings"?

et's engage in some wild generalization and divide humanity into two factions: deaf and non-deaf. The non-deaf people constitute the majority; the deaf people, the minority. Any majority group uses terms to describe themselves (insiders) and the minority (outsiders). Conversely, the minority, which sees *themselves* as insiders, uses its own terms to describe the majority (outsiders). Deaf people commonly use the term *hearing* (singular noun) or *hearings* (plural noun) to describe the non-deaf majority. As used by deaf people, it means "people who can hear," i.e., non-deaf. The word "hearing" is, of course, found in the dictionary, meaning "the capacity to hear" or "the range of audibility." But this particular usage is not. It's a specifically Deaf usage. As such, it may come as a shock to some non-deaf folks.

Non-deaf people—that is, people with normal hearing—don't think of themselves as being "hearing." They take their normal hearing for granted, as they do their other faculties. *Hearing* is a term employed by the deaf outsiders, applied to the non-deaf insiders. This kind of label can make the "labelee" uncomfortable.

How important are labels? Our long and bitter experience as an oppressed minority group has shown that labels can be very powerful weapons. Labels have caused us an immeasurable amount of damage—in terms of self-esteem, pride, and squelched potential, as well as the more tangible economic sense. The labels that have been applied to deaf people throughout the millennia have called attention to our supposed deficits—"deaf-and-dumb," "deaf-mute," "deaf and mute," "mute," etc.—never our strengths. These labels emphasize our apparent freakishness, not our normality. No member of the majority culture would endure labels like these, calling into question their very ability to *think*. So here we have a case of the tables being turned. Deaf people, seeing their own deafness as a normal characteristic, much like an ethnic identity, see the non-deaf majority as the outsiders, the different ones, the people who lack a Deaf identity. They use the indispensable term *hearing*. It's not necessarily a pejorative term (after all, once upon a time "deaf-and-dumb" was a placidly neutral expression), but it can be employed as a weapon, a put-down.

The sign for *hearing* is an extended index finger making a quick repeated horizontal rolling motion in front of the mouth, symbolizing speaking-with-the-voice. Communicating with hearing people, deaf people occasionally use the term *hearie*. The sign is made like *hearing*. *Hearie* can be used as a term of insult applied to one hearing person, or can refer to a group of hearing people, or society (the "Hearing" culture) in its most general sense. *Hearing* can describe attitudes, mindsets, lifestyles, values, even culinary preferences. (As in **Children of a Lesser God**, when Orin calls veal piccata and sushi "*'hearing'* food"). Familiar Deaf expressions of exasperation are "They're just a bunch of hearings" or

"What do you expect from hearings?" Then there's the ultimate expression of prejudice: "I don't like hearings."

A new term, *hearo* (or *hear-o*), describes a deaf person who apes hearing people.* The sign for *hear-o* is literally "hearing-in-the-head"—shifting the *hearing/hearie* sign from the mouth to the forehead. The sign itself has been in currency for some time. (It's analogous to a Black person calling another Black person an "Oreo"—Black on the outside, white inside.) *Hear-o* is an equally pejorative term. Whether or not you find it amusing depends on your point of view.

Aren't these labels insulting? Not necessarily—they reflect a normal human trait of expressing belonging to a group and distinguishing ourselves from those who are different. The terms used by deaf people to insult or poke fun at the hearing majority cannot compare with the nastiness of the terms the hearing majority has long used against us.

*And remember, folks, you read it here first!

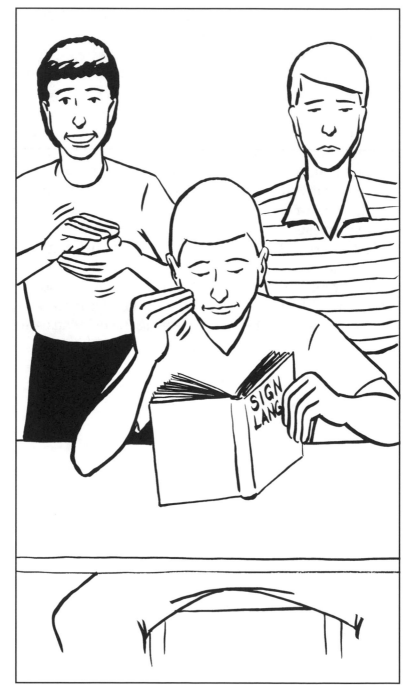

Chapter 50

In my pamphlets and textbooks, Deaf people are portrayed as being delighted when "the Hearing" learn Signing. But I get the impression from other sources that Deaf people resent hearing people doing that. What's the real situation?

t depends on what your motivation is in learning how to Sign, your attitude, the context, who's teaching you, who's learning with you, and who you're mingling with. Some Deaf people consider themselves guardians of Deaf culture, an embattled way of life, and are fiercely protective of ASL. They seek to "preserve the purity" of the language, which has been becoming increasingly "polluted" by "foreign" intrusions such as Manually Coded English (MCE).*

ASL is a living language, and like any other living language, it is subject to change. It is constantly evolving. (Remember how incensed some conservative French citizens were by the influx of Americanisms like *le weekend, le drugstore, le caddy, le hot dog,* and *les blue jeans*?) ASL, too, is constantly picking up and trying on "foreign loan words." Fad signs appear, blaze briefly, and die out. New signs are constantly being devised to keep pace with technology and the news. All go through a sifting process—the useful ones are retained, obsolete ones dropped.

There is, however, a difference between influences "naturally" picked up and shared among Deaf peers, and artificial constructions—"to be" forms, initialized signs like "doctor" with a "d," and notorious suffixes like "-ness" and the participle "-ing"—which are imposed from without, namely by hearing (and some deaf) educators. Many Deaf people (by no means extremists) feel that such intrusions degrade the beauty of ASL. Keep in mind that ASL is the one thing Deaf people here can truly call their own. It is the precious inheritance of the Deaf community, passed from parent to child, or more commonly, child to child. It has survived the efforts of "well-meaning" oralists to wipe it out. Its users have experienced the terrible humiliation of being robbed of their language. Many older Deaf people recall how they were forbidden to Sign in class or public, punished for being caught Signing, forced to Sign on the sly. Now that we are experiencing a great flowering of ASL artistry—theatre, poetry, sign mime, storytelling, religious signing—there is an understandable fear that "the Hearing" are going to try to take it over and wrest it from its rightful possessors.

Deaf citizens rightfully resent hearing people's learning ASL so they can take over agencies serving Deaf people—in other words, take Deaf people's jobs away while increasing their own power in the Deaf community. We feel that there is no shortage of qualified Deaf candidates for such jobs, and that since hearing people have an unlimited choice of jobs elsewhere, our preference is for Deaf people themselves to coordinate the agencies that benefit their own community. That's hardly a snobbish attitude. Deaf people, after all, are still barred from many positions. Learning someone else's native language in order to enhance one's own personal power and make money from their community is a form of exploitation we're all familiar with.

There is nothing intrinsically immoral about a hearing person's learning ASL to fulfill a foreign-language requirement or so s/he can better communicate with Deaf friends, co-workers, etc. It can be a wonderful thing. But Deaf people rightfully resent the attitude 'I'm going to become fluent in Sign so I can *help* the Deaf, *interpret* for them, *save* them.' Some interpreters *are* good; some are *bad*. Look at it this way: to some Deaf people, an interpreter is a hearing person who earns money off Deaf people's language. Who earns more—interpreters or the Deaf people who teach them ASL? (Clue: An interpreter can earn as much as $50 an hour; an ASL teacher, as little as $3 an hour. And who enjoys the proceeds of ASL books published by mainstream publishers? Hearing or Deaf?)

Many feel that ASL belongs to Deaf people, period. It may be shared but not owned by others. They resent the idea of hearing people messing with their language. And you can't blame them for that.

---

*According to Dr. Robert Panara, the distinguished Deaf professor, scholar, and author, the "Combined Method" (classroom signing) has long included ASL and MCE. "Signed English was the mainstay method at Gallaudet and Schools for the Deaf all during the years 1880 to today in the attempt to combat and counteract Oralism."

Chapter 51

Why don't some deaf people trust hearing people?

et's rephrase the question: *Why don't some black people trust white people?* The memories of slavery, oppression, violence, discrimination, denial of opportunities. Through the centuries, deaf people have likewise been victims of oppression, although, we admit, we have never been kidnapped from our native countries and forced *en masse* into slavery. The discrimination we have faced is of a subtler variety, although more ancient. Another substitution: *Why don't some (Native) American Indians trust white people?* Like American Indian children, our Deaf ancestors were denied access to their native language, and forced to assimilate into an alien (majority) culture. Even if they tried to behave and talk like the majority, they weren't really accepted.

Worthy of mention here, too, is the fact that hearing people in abundance have the jobs which deaf people feel are rightfully theirs, particularly in the areas of education and human services. Deaf people generally have needs and interests unique to themselves which can be most effectively addressed by themselves.

Traditionally, Deaf people have been looked upon as "different." As with any cultural minority, perhaps more so, there has been a strong "huddling instinct"— Deaf people banding together and giving each other support and sympathy, keeping ASL alive, and not having any more to do with the outside (Hearing) culture than is necessary. You don't have to be a whiz in sociology to recognize that Deaf people have been op-pressed for centuries. Negative views of deafness (and the abilities of deaf people) are at least as old as Aristotle—no doubt older. And with such oppression have come ignorance, misunderstandings, and hostility, all of which are, unfortunately, still far too prevalent.

We have already mentioned several times the old campaign against ASL in the deaf schools. The tide is turning, but immeasurable damage has been done. Deaf adults still recall some of their teachers, the oppressive influence of these powerful ambassadors of Hearing culture. They look back with anger. As recently as our grandparents' and parents' generations, deaf children were taught that deafness was bad, Signing was not socially acceptable, something that had to be hidden, as if it was shameful and dirty, and that, if they wanted to achieve Acceptance, Happiness, and Fulfillment, they should act as "Hearing" as possible.

These negative attitudes have largely given way to more positive views, but the memory remains. In some cases, oppression of deaf children isn't just a memory; it's still happening. Certain groups of hearing people still oppress Deaf people. They want to suppress ASL. They threaten Deaf people.

Some older Deaf people have vivid memories of being taken advantage of by unscrupulous hearing salesmen and agents who sold them appliances, furniture, or automobiles on the installment plan and "conned" them into signing contracts whose fine print they didn't un-derstand. The result? The items they thought they owned were repossessed. All that was gained was a bitter education in the less admirable ways of the Hearing world.

Old prejudices and cultural attitudes die hard. Most Deaf people *are* willing to meet the Hearing community halfway. If the Hearing community really wants to establish mutual trust, it must be able to convince the Deaf community that it has its welfare at heart. But there must be open communication and genuine respect. No more "plantation mentality;" no more paternalism. The recent threatend closings of Deaf schools, which strikes at the very heart of Deaf culture, do not bode well.

Chapter 52

What do you mean,
"An interpreter is a person
who earns money off
Deaf people's language"?!

ntil the mid-1960s, there was no such thing as professional interpreters. Interpreting was not a profession; it was a favor hearing children did for their Deaf parents, or hearing parents did for their Deaf children. A skilled hearing relative or neighbor could be pressed into service when needed—if a Deaf person had to consult with a lawyer or doctor, etc. It was an amateur's field. There was no code of ethics, no standards, no certifying process.

In 1964, the Registry of Interpreters for the Deaf, the national certifying body, was founded. With the recognition of interpreting as a profession, our social status has changed tremendously—for the better. To keep pace with the increasing demand, more and more interpreters are being trained and certified. (The Americans with Disabilities Act will certainly encourage the profession even further.) Interpreters have become a fact of life, a part of the American scene. Switch on the evening news, and wherever you see a Presidential candidate or governmental bigwig addressing a crowd, there's usually an interpreter just to the side of the podium. Some hearing theatergoers, even those who feel that theatrical interpreters are distracting, a visual annoyance, may find themselves taking a peek—they're curious, even fascinated. The public visibility of interpreters has certainly fostered new awareness of Deaf people, their language, and their needs.

Interpreting has become a respectable, if tough and occasionally hazardous, profession. Its rigid code of ethics was designed to protect the privacy of both parties, but it can work against the Deaf client. In a courtroom setting, an interpreter is forbidden to explain ANYTHING to the jury, even if they're prejudiced against the Deaf person. We've read the harrowing account of a brilliant hearing woman, a native Signer, daughter of Deaf parents, recalling her stint as a city-appointed interpreter in the courtroom and at a psychiatric clinic. She felt terribly constrained by the code of ethics; although she wanted to, she was forbidden to explain to the jurors why her client, a young, poor Black woman who killed her sister's boyfriend in self-defense, was acting the way she did. She made clicking and grunting noises as she gave her testimony in Sign. This defendant didn't *know* that she was making these "weird" sounds, but they helped to prejudice the jury against her. She was found guilty of first-degree murder and sentenced to a stiff prison term. The interpreter, who sympathized with the woman, was helpless to aid her in court.

In the days of "Mom 'n' Pop" interpreters, the Deaf client wasn't expected to pay a fee. It was a favor rendered by family or a friend. With the rise of professional interpreters, a Deaf person who needs an interpreter (say, to consult a lawyer) often has to foot the bill. The cost of an interpreter is as high as $50 an hour. Who pays? We do, often. A good number of Deaf people cannot afford to hire an interpreter.

Where do interpreters learn their trade? They take courses. Who teaches them? Very often, native-ASL users, Deaf people. How much do these teachers earn per hour? We have it on good authority (from an actual sign-language instructor) that a high-school teacher may earn as little as $5-$7 per hour while a college-level teacher will do better—$15-$30 per hour. (It depends on the setting.) And how much do interpreters earn? Unlike teachers, they have the power to set their own fees. They generally earn $30-$50 per hour.

A few things to keep in mind: Freelance interpreters (who command those $30-to-$50-per-hour sums) may not work full-time (i.e., 40 hours a week). Their interpreting schedules may be notably irregular, as few as 10 hours a week. (Thirty hours a week is considered exceptionally good for a freelancer.) So a freelancer generally puts in fewer hours than a staff interpreter in an educational setting who works or is on call full-time (say, between 20 and 40 hours a week). They may be earning pretty much the same as a sign-language instructor ($15-$30 per hour)—some even less.

Moreover, the majority of students in interpreter-training programs pay their own way. In some colleges, ITP tuition is steep. Like many other students, they take out loans to meet the high cost of their education. Very few get scholarships.

Well, you may say, interpreting is a physically and mentally challenging, frequently exhausting, field demanding a high level of skill. Well, we reply, the same can be said of sign-language instructors. So why do interpreters earn $30 to $50 an hour while the people who teach them earn $5 to $15 per hour?

Could it be that teaching just doesn't command the same prestige as interpreting? Teaching is expected to be a "labor of love." Interpreting is a profession. Most interpreters enter the profession because it's a good career, not necessarily because they love ASL or cherish Deaf culture. The more professional distance between the interpreter and client, the better. Some Deaf people, seeing how much money interpreters make (especially compared to their teachers), resent it. (Imagine how you'd feel, knowing that the graduates will always earn more—in some cases, a lot more—than those who teach them. How many administrators are willing to pay a teacher $30 or $50 an hour? Yet an interpreter can demand—and receive—high fees.)

Any hearing person can become an interpreter. The job market is open to all hearing people. It is *not* open to all Deaf people. (They are severely limited in the kind of interpreting they can do: sign-to-sign.) So you have a corps of hearing people earning money off Deaf people's sign language—a profession more or less off-limits to Deaf people themselves.

Even so, some interpreters (and a few sign-language teachers) donate their services to the Deaf community— free of charge, that is.

An interpreter who "slips" can create costly misunderstandings or cause considerable damage to the client. An interpreter who makes a mistake while interpreting a Deaf person's testimony in court can have a destructive effect on his or her life. A *few* interpreters like to play God over their clients. They're power-hungry; they enjoy the feeling of controlling Deaf people.

That said, we'd like to emphasize that there are a few truly superb interpreters. They respect Deaf people; they have a good attitude towards Deaf culture and sign language. They charge reasonable rates. In return, they are respected and esteemed by the Deaf community. *And* there are a few truly bad interpreters—the ones who cause trouble for their profession by "giving interpreters a bad name." The majority of interpreters are in between. They're in a career; they earn money.

If you have difficulty understanding why we made

our statement about interpreters in the first place, why not ask a Deaf person how s/he feels about interpreters? Chances are, they'll echo some of the things we're saying here.

Chapter 53

In our city it seems that the churches are beginning to reach out to the Deaf community. Is this the case in other parts of the U.S.?

The National Information Center on Deafness referred this question to Duane King of Deaf Missions (Council Bluffs, Iowa). His response:

es, more hearing churches do seem to be reaching out to deaf people. That is certainly not to say that enough of the reaching-out is done in the right way. Even so, it is encouraging to me to see the reaching-out happening.

As you must know, a very large percentage of the culturally-Deaf people are virtually untouched by most of the reaching-out that is done by hearing churches. The ordinary interpreted service does not appeal to a person for whom English is a foreign language. But I feel that, more and more, the hearing churches are beginning to realize the need for Deaf people to have worship and study and fellowship that is led by Deaf people, and primarily prepared for Deaf people. It might be [possible] someday (far in the future, I'm afraid) that you would ask another question: "Do more Deaf churches seem to be reaching out to hearing people?!"

Even though more hearing churches do seem to be reaching out to Deaf people, an ironic turn of events seems to be making it so that some Deaf people (often influenced by hearing people who are strongly supportive of Deaf culture) are refusing to be touched, even though someone is reaching out to them. The current trend toward separation of cultures, or at least the restoration of Deaf culture, naturally leads one to the conclusion that to reach people of the Deaf Culture, we must train a Deaf person who will be accepted by the culture. Whether or not this is right, it is a fact of the 1990s.

Of course, this is one person's point of view. There must be many other opinions!

▲ ▲ ▲

Church Outreach: a few comments of our own

The relationship between the church and deaf education is quite old. The earliest deaf children known to receive an education were from wealthy and aristocratic 16th-century Spanish families whose parents sent them to monasteries (to keep them out of society and to prevent them from reproducing). Our commonly used manual alphabet is based one used in 16th-century Spain. It was evidently borrowed from the monastic practice of communicating in silence and was adapted for use with deaf pupils.

The Abbé de l'Epée and Thomas Hopkins Gallaudet both had religious missions—to educate the deaf to enable them to attain salvation. The Institut National in Paris was Catholic, as the Hartford Asylum was Congregationalist. Gallaudet's eldest son, Thomas, became an Episcopalian priest. He founded the first Deaf congregation in the States, St. Ann's Church for the Deaf, in

Manhattan. He is credited with introducing Signed religious services. Largely because of his work, the Episcopalian Church took the lead in Deaf outreach.

And it should be noted that the church, by offering signed Sunday services, helped keep ASL alive during the "dark ages" of oralism. Religious signing can be extraordinarily beautiful and uplifting.

Today, the U.S. Catholic Church has a Deaf outreach program, administering several schools for the deaf. (Some are oral; some signing.)

There are a few Jewish synagogues for Deaf congregations, primarily in California and New York. Because of the relatively tiny Jewish deaf population (and de-emphasis on missionizing), outreach is on a much smaller scale than among Catholics or Protestants. There are clubs and organizations for Jewish Deaf people, but no Jewish day schools that use sign language.

There is one branch of a certain fundamentalist Christian church that specializes in missionary outreach to deaf people. Some of us find this practice disturbing, as this church places great emphasis on "hell" and "eternal damnation." We feel that the missionaries are out to collect as many Deaf souls as they can, so they can gain credit for "saving the Deaf." They prey on naïve Deaf people who have never had a religious education, and who sometimes "fall for it." These people join the church not from interest or gratitude, but out of fear. Once in the church, they are effectively brainwashed. This church preaches a gospel of narrow-minded intolerance towards Jews and other non-Christians (i.e., Catholics). Yet it maintains an active presence in our community. We consider this spiritual exploitation—ancient oppression in new religious trappings.

Chapter 54

"How do deaf people feel when a hearing person approaches them in public using sign language?"

My question is: How do deaf people feel when a hearing person approaches them in public using their language? Example: I'm in line at the store and I notice two deaf people busy in conversation. I've never met them before but I'd love to say hello and find out more about them. Almost always I never do for fear I'll come across sounding paternalistic: "Hi, I can help you, I can interpret for you," or bragging: "Hi, I know what you're saying and these poor hearing people don't."

I believe my motives are pure. I'm fascinated with your language, culture and history but really I don't know what to say, or **shouldn't** say in these situations. Thank you.

A. C.
Granada Hills, California

 t's perfectly OK to be fascinated by Deaf culture and the way Deaf people communicate, and quite understandable to be intrigued by seeing them signing in public. But when it comes to a hearing stranger joining in their conversation with an offer to "interpret" or to "help," some Deaf people are going to resent it, and may react with embarrassment and annoyance. If Deaf people need help with interpreting, *they* will ask for it. Offers of help, however well-intentioned, are seen as patronizing, perpetuating an offensive stereotype of Deaf people as helpless and vulnerable.

To approach or not to approach? This question is widely discussed among Deaf people. Some like the idea; some do not.

As for letting Deaf people know that you enjoy their language, it's all common sense. Whether or not to greet them depends on the setting. For example, if the Deaf people are in line at a bank or store, it's best not to say anything, as they're preoccupied, busy, or in a hurry. If, however, you see Signers at a bus stop or sitting near you in the bus, it's OK to say "Hello, how are you?", as there are fewer distractions. Just remember not to control the conversation. Let them control it.

One sure-fire "ice-breaker" is to ask the Deaf person, "What school did you go to?" Deaf people love to talk about their old schools—their experiences, their teachers, their favorite classes and activities, the bad stuff (maybe), sports, friends, where their schoolmates are now. Deaf people, it seems, meeting each other for the first time, never fail to exchange and compare school experiences. It's a passionately cherished topic. You can also ask, "What year did you graduate?" and "Did you go to college?" The Deaf person may give you a run-down of her/his experiences—which are most likely worth listening to—and quite possibly afford you some insight into the Deaf experience in general.

Be prepared to answer some questions yourself. When Deaf people meet a signing hearing person, they will usually ask right away, "Where did you learn sign language from?" Answer promptly—and be honest. Suppose you say, "Oh, I took a series of classes at the Centerville Community College." They will then ask, "Who was your teacher?" If you studied with a good Deaf teacher, or a hearing teacher who is respected in the

Deaf community, so much the better.

Needless to say, the more skillful your signing (receptive and expressive), the better your chance of establishing a friendly conversation. Deaf people find it particularly annoying when hearing strangers come over, acting "chummy," mangled fingerspelling and butchered signs flying off their hands.

Chapter 55

"I understand it is bad manners to watch people Signing without their knowing that you also Sign. But is it bad manners to interrupt people who are Signing and telling them that you are taking courses in ASL even if you sign in English?"

I understand it is bad manners to watch people signing without their knowing that you also Sign. But there's always that tendency for a student to see if you can understand anything. Is it bad manners to interrupt such people and tell them that you are taking courses in ASL even if you sign in English?

I'm writing this in response to an article our ASL teacher gave us, reprinted from **DEAF LIFE**, "ASL: What is it?" [See Chapter 1.] And as it says, ASL is a beautiful and expressive language and a pleasure to learn and observe.

Thanks for your time and help.

R. M.
Wheaton, Maryland

 or all practical purposes, there is no such thing as a "private" ASL conversation in public—that is, within eyeshot of other people. What two Deaf people are discussing is out in the open for everyone else to see. Signs can be read straight across a crowded room, a campus quad, or from a window several stories up! Signing conversationalists in a "Voice" environment rely on the non-comprehension of the surrounding hearing crowd to safeguard the confidentiality of their talk—that is, they assume that since nobody else will understand what they're talking about, they're "protected." Anyone who wants to have a private talk in an "ASL" environment (such as the Gallaudet campus) has to duck behind the shrubbery, use a jacket as a "sign-shield" (holding the jacket out with one hand, signing with the other), or adopt a smaller, discreetly formed, disguised style of Signing which snoopers will find harder to read—the visual equivalent of a whisper. In some public Signing environments, like a college cafeteria, club, lobby, or bus, it's fair game to watch others Signing, and to join in.

It's *not* bad manners to enter a conversation, but it shouldn't be an intrusion. It all depends on the situation and who you're with. You have to ascertain the mood of the interchange—if it's casual and relaxed, chit-chat style, and you're reasonably certain the Deaf people will accept your presence, you can draw near, wait for a suitable opening, gesture/wave for attention (or use the gentle shoulder-pat approach), and sign, "Oh, you're Deaf? Ah, good! I know some sign language," or "Hello, I saw you signing. I'm taking an ASL class now," or the like. Be prepared to introduce yourself; fingerspell your name, and give your name-sign.* The more skillful your Signing is, the easier it will be for you. There's no real way to predict how others will react. Some will undoubtedly be warm, bemused. Others may give you the "freeze-out" treatment. Use your intuition and play it by eye.

Let the others control the conversation. You can make a learning game of it—see how much you understand, if you can keep up with the lightning pace of ASL interchanges—*if* they continue using ASL near you. Deaf people will often politely "code-switch" to Pidgin Sign English to make it easier for the hearing participant or onlooker, so it isn't at all easy for hearing persons to drop by and watch an ASL interchange at close range, and to participate.

*Deaf people meeting each other for the first time will often converse for 5 or 10 minutes, then exchange their names (fingerspelled, with name-signs) before they part.

Chapter 56

I've noticed that when someone uses the ILY sign in public, some of my Deaf friends have dismayed expressions on their faces. Don't they like it?

he best-known Deaf sign isn't strictly ASL, but a combination of three letters of the standard American-European manual alphabet: I, L, and Y (i.e., I Love You). Bend your middle and ring fingers into your palm, extend pinkie, index, and thumb, turn your palm outwards, and you have it.

For all its newfound popularity, the ILY sign has been around for nearly a century. **Deaf Heritage** has traced it as far back as 1905. If so, it fell into disuse, but evidently was never entirely forgotten. However, many of those who attended schools for the deaf during the 1960s and 1970s don't recall seeing an ILY *anywhere*. It achieved "star exposure" in the mid-70s after Presidential candidate Jimmy Carter picked it up from a group of Deaf supporters in the Midwest. (His predecessor, Gerald Ford, had also learned it from Deaf people.) During his famous inaugural walk down Pennsylvania Avenue (most other presidents rode grandly in a limousine), Carter was photographed flashing the ILY to a group of Deaf people on the sidewalk. These photos, front-page-style, were published in the national media. Deaf people, who recognized the sign immediately, were delighted. Instant fame for the ILY.

That was in 1977. Since then, it seems, everyone's gotten into the act. We've seen ILYs on the national news (video footage from Operation Desert Storm showed an American soldier on a tank, triumphantly flashing it), all over the place. Deaf people and their hearing friends have made the ILY arguably the best-known handsign in the world (competing in popularity with the classic "V-for-victory"). It's even been used to summon help. Some years back, we read an account of a deaf couple whose car broke down on a highway. They stood by their disabled car, trying to flag down passing motorists, without luck. Then they thought of trying the ILY. It worked. A truck whizzed by them, then braked, backed up, and pulled over. It turned out that the folks who owned the truck had a young daughter who watched *Sesame Street*, and had picked up the ILY sign from series regular Linda Bove. When she saw the couple standing by their car bravely flashing the ILY, she cried, "Daddy, stop! Those people are deaf, and they need help!" And the girl's father did stop. Help came.

And so the ILY has become the best-known symbol of the Deaf community. In catalogues specializing in Deaf-oriented products, you can find ILY charms, vases, mugs, keychains, stickers, magnets, figurines, and T-shirts. Some deaf (and hearing) people love the ILY so much that they avidly collect ILY paraphernalia—much as others collect Barbie dolls, Grateful Dead mementos, or knickknacks representing their sign of the zodiac.

In the process, an intimate, tender sign has lost most of its original force and virtually all significance. What was once a charming and concise way to say "I love you" now means "Hiya."

The ILY has become so popular and widespread, so ubiquitous, that it's become a visual cliché—the "Smiley Face" of Deaf Culture. What we have is a case of overkill.

And with overexposure comes abuse. You can find hearing people who have no previous acquaintance with Deaf people or sign language (and no intention of learning more about either), giddily flashing the ILY at every deaf person (or every person they *think* is deaf) whom they run across. Sometimes these well-meaning folks aren't even making the handsign correctly. (Do it wrong and you generally end up with the sign for "bullshit"—not the sort of thing you'd want to wave at a stranger.)* It's as though these people think the "ILY" is the be-all and end-all of Deaf-Hearing communication, some kind of magic catchword. Once they learn the ILY, they're OK with deaf people, they're safe. No wonder that some deaf people react with quizzical expressions. They're thinking, "What's up with this one?!"

Among Deaf people, it's acceptable to flash the ILY at another person from a distance, as it shows up well. It *is* considered gauche to flash the ILY at close range. If an uninformed hearing person walks into a gathering of Deaf people and cheerily waves the ILY, s/he had better be prepared for some sour looks!

Some of us love the ILY; some tolerate it; some are sick of it. (To some, it's not cute anymore, just corny.) Some Deaf people hate the ILY, really loathe it. It makes them shudder to see it, and they have to repress a momentary urge to thwack ILY-flashers off their feet. That could account for those dismayed expressions you've seen. They're restraining themselves.

*This is what happened to the unfortunate Vice President Walter Mondale during that same Inauguration Day parade. **Deaf Heritage** describes how Mondale, "following [Carter] in an open car, unfamiliar with the symbol, but gamely trying to respond to the same group [of Deaf well-wishers], was seen innocently waving an obscene gesture!" (Chapter 15, p. 373)

Chapter 57

If there is a Hearing speaker, the Deaf audience claps their hands. If there is a Deaf speaker, the Deaf audience waves their hands. But if there is a Deaf speaker and a Hearing audience who know little or nothing about Deaf culture, what should they do?

H.R.
Columbia, Maryland

embers of any audience where there is a Deaf speaker or performer *should* applaud by waving their hands, "Deaf-Culture" style. It's a matter of simple courtesy. If they applaud by clapping their hands in the conventional "Hearing" fashion, the Deaf speaker will probably *see* it and appreciate the thought—but waving-hands applause will have so much more impact and be all the more appreciated. If the intention (applause) is genuine, why not choose the vehicle that can express it most powerfully? For us, waving hands carries better. And it's not difficult to do.

When we wish to honor people of a different culture, we do it by expressing our esteem for them in their own language—or, at least, in terms they can understand. By waving their hands, Hearing audiences show that they recognize and respect the Deaf speaker as a person.

Variously known as "Deaf applause," "visual applause," or "flying hands," an audience's waving hands, hats, or handkerchiefs to signal its appreciation of a Deaf person is really an old practice, undoubtedly invented and re-invented through the centuries on the spur of the moment. There are published allusions to it going back to the mid-19th century—and we will likely uncover even earlier ones. We see these as a tribute to human ingenuity in overcoming a communication barrier.

In **DEAF LIFE**, we've noted an 1892 description of spectators at a Washington, D.C. baseball field, delighted by the exploits of Deaf outfielder William Ellsworth "Dummy" Hoy, rising up *en masse* and "wildly waving hats and arms." Readers have shared with us a mid-19th-century reference to an audience's waving their handkerchiefs to the late-deafened Czech composer Bedrich Smetana; a 1912 report in **The Silent Worker** of an audience at the Chautauqua Institute applauding a Deaf presenter by similarly waving handkerchiefs (the "Chautauqua Salute"); and a firsthand account of a Deaf slo-pitch softball team from Edmonton, Alberta, who waved hotel dinner napkins at an awards banquet (1980), sparking a visual-applause trend in Canada. Participants in the National Festival of Arts of the Deaf, also in Alberta (1984), were even issued "clapkerchiefs"—little pieces of imprinted cloth to be used for applauding. Those who forgot to bring them waved their hands in the air.

Likewise, "waving hands" seems to have caught on in France around the same time and spread through the Deaf community there; some U.S. visitors saw it in 1985 and brought it back. By the time of The DEAF WAY International Conference and Festival (Washington, D.C., July 1989), everybody seemed to be doing it. It spread like the proverbial wildfire because it was easy, fun, and foolproof. It makes a striking scene—even a beautiful one.

Deaf applause suits our visual orientation precisely. It doesn't demand unusual exertion (unlike clapping and shouting, which can leave you with sore hands or a hoarse throat). Any audience can clap politely (even if they're bored), but waving hands does demand kinetic participation—you *really* have to get into it, show spirit. But what better way to do it? To a Deaf person facing such an audience, a forest of waving hands is a glorious sight.

References:

"The Colorful Legacy of 'Dummy' Hoy," **DEAF LIFE**, November 1992, p. 22. The reference is to a remark by Henry Furness in **Sporting Life**, 1892: "When outfielder Hoy made a brilliant catch, the crowd arose *en masse* and wildly waved hats and arms. It was the only way in which they could testify their appreciation to the deaf-mute athlete."

Bummy Burstein, "The Saga of the Waving Applause," **DEAF LIFE**, July 1992, pp. 26-27.

"Waving hands: a Canadian perspective," letter by Roger J. Carver, M.Ed., **DEAF LIFE**, October 1992, p. 6.

"The 'Chautauqua Salute,'" letter by Harry Lang, **DEAF LIFE**, December 1992, p. 4.

Chapter 58

"Should my office clerks be given different, lesser duties because they are deaf?"

Two deaf clerks work for me. One was born deaf, we'll call her "D." The other had spoken and knew English before becoming deaf; we'll call her "L." "L" is obviously intelligent. She often intimidates "D." Perhaps it's "L's" culture, but she even "said" to me, "I *demand* . . ." "D" has her good qualities but is not "obviously intelligent." She forgets easily. For instance, we get batches of work in the unit. They are numbered with batch numbers. They are supposed to be logged onto a log each day. "D" often forgets to. We have work to control onto computer terminals; neither "D" nor "L" remembers all steps even though they have books and their own notes.

"D" does not understand English very well. I can't sign. "D" is the permanent clerk, "L" is the "helper." However, "L" interprets for "D" and often acts superior.

I know I must learn to sign. This doesn't happen overnight. I sometimes get very frustrated.

Should these clerks be given different, lesser duties because they are deaf? Does being deaf hinder them from performing daily tasks the same as the other clerks?

Any understanding you can give me will be greatly appreciated.

S. S.
Cumming, Georgia

o start with, let's do a bit of sweeping-up of some "sweeping generalizations." We can start with such nuggets of wisdom as 'Deaf workers can't handle abstract thinking as well as hearing can'; 'Deaf workers have difficulty remembering daily tasks'; 'Deaf workers just aren't as attentive to detail'; 'Deaf workers can't understand English', etc., etc., etc. That's bad logic and bad politics.

Is it a matter of intelligence? Education? Aptitude, perhaps? We *will* venture to say that deafness is most likely *not* to blame. This may not be much of a consolation, but it's probably the truth. Deafness has nothing to do with disorganization or forgetfulness.

Your two troublesome clerks, "D" and "L," could just as well be hearing. ('But of course,' you may say, 'if they were hearing, there'd *be* no problem!') Let's hypothesize (and exaggerate) a bit. We all know of office clerks with perfect hearing who were unsuccessful at carrying out their tasks—poor performers, sloppy, careless, forgetful, mentally disorganized, bad attitudes—or any combination of these. I'm sure that plenty of supervisors have gotten two under-performers at the same time who work (and forget) together and set up a pecking order of sorts. Can we blame their incompetence on the fact that they're hearing?

Now, you suggest that "D" and "L" have some good qualities—enough to make you hesitate before booting them down the ladder. However, the current situation is hurting the company—work not logged in, directions forgotten, tasks not completed properly. What to do?

Before reassigning (demoting?) "D" or "L," you might want to attack the memory problem. Evidently "D" and "L" have difficulty remembering/completing tasks, even with their own notes. Take a positive approach. Since Deaf people tend to have a strong visual sense, you might try making a few "constant reminders"—bold, colorful flow-charts or stand-up desk cards listing your workers' responsibilities ("Every day: Log on such-and-such"). Post them in full sight of their workstations (where their eyes will *have* to keep lighting on them). You could even make laminated ones that they *have* to check off, task by task, using water-soluble or china markers. See if that helps.

"D,"who doesn't understand English very well, is in roughly the same position as a native speaker of Chinese whose grasp of a second language, English, just isn't very advanced. And your grasp of her native language—well, it isn't there yet. ("L" is "post-lingually deafened," so her frustrations are different. In a sense, she's "stuck" between you and "D.")

We encourage you to start learning sign language as a step towards establishing a truly bilingual workplace. Maybe your signing—or seeing that you're making a genuine commitment to learning Sign—will help "D" and "L" understand and cooperate. If you can't learn Sign fast, use plenty of body language. Point with your finger. Be expressive. Be visual.

In response to your final question, we want to stress that deafness need not be a hindrance to clerical compe-tence, a retentive memory, abstract thinking, quality performance, or excellence in general. What Deaf people are fighting for is not preferential treatment, unearned breaks, or the soft life. Our goal is to be capable of functioning in the world, in whatever path we choose, doing our best at what we do best, judged by our true abilities, and standing on our own strengths. The same as with hearing professionals. We expect no less of ourselves than the world expects of any professionals. That's our idea of *real* equality.

Chapter 59

Do Deaf people ever wish they were hearing?

es, primarily because they are disgusted with having to deal with the constant bullshit they get from the hearing world—restrictions, discrimination, *can't* this, *can't* that. *And* the peculiar brand of bullshit found in the Deaf community—the gossip, the backstabbing.

Do Deaf people suffer from sensory deprivation? Most don't. Surprisingly, many born-deaf people don't "miss" sound, music, and spoken conversation anywhere near as much as hearing people think they do. They don't find themselves missing what they never had. (Similarly, many people who are born blind or early-blinded, when asked if they don't miss the beauties of the visual world, colors, rainbows, and sunsets, have said that they can't miss something they've never experienced.) Late-deafened people are a different matter entirely.* They've lost an integral aspect of their lives they've taken for granted (as do hearing people), and their feelings of loss and pain should never be denigrated. Born-deaf adults, as a rule, tend to be well-adjusted, with a positive view of themselves as Deaf people. They see themselves as whole persons, *not* broken ears, *not* defective hearing machines, *not* deprived of "normalcy." If they don't miss the beauties of music (and, of course, it depends on what you mean by *music*), it's because they have other things going on in their heads and their lives that keep them occupied.

Occasionally, hearing people tell us how much they

"envy" the supposed peace and quiet which (they imagine) deaf people experience in their "silent world." An understandable, but patronizing sentiment. Our lives are filled with hubbub and noise—visual noise—and we're discriminated against. (We pay a pretty high price for that "peace and quiet.")

A good number of Deaf people don't see the spoken word as the supreme unit of communication. Their early experiences with speech may not be pleasant or productive. They have a fully-developed, subtle, and expressive means of communication—sign language—which suits their needs perfectly. Sometimes they feel a bit sorry for hearing people who can't sign. Signing adds visual zip to one's life—why would *anyone* want to be without it?

One of the worst things about being deaf is the isolation we experience—which has nothing to do with the quality of our residual hearing and much to do with the quality of social attitudes. A problem frequently experienced by oral and mainstreamed deaf children is the absence of deaf adult mentors (a.k.a. "role models"). A number of these deaf children honestly believe that they're going to become hearing when they grow up. Since they're surrounded by hearing teachers, therapists, counselors, and staffers, and since their families and all other adults they meet are hearing, they logically assume that there are no deaf adults in the world, and therefore, once they reach adulthood, they too will be hearing. This is one reason why so many mainstreamed deaf children have "difficulties adjusting." It simply underscores the vital need to bring successful deaf/Deaf adults into these children's lives.

Anyone who has grown up in the Deaf community knows that Deaf people can be unbelievably vicious to other Deaf people—especially those whose only crime is to be "different," to aspire to something which is not the "norm," to cherish a "hearing" ambition, and to succeed in it. Deaf people trashing other Deaf people is a shameful fact of life for many of us. It originates in jealousy. Instead of encouragement and support, achievers get sneers. Instead of appreciation (let alone admiration), backstabbing. Instead of understanding, hostility. Add this to the "Hearing" discrimination and incomprehension they are already battling, and you have a pretty heavy burden, one that can be intolerable. Thus, a number of Deaf people have to deal—simultaneously—with bullshit from both Hearing and Deaf communities. Small wonder that some creative Deaf people who have labored diligently to increase understanding and acceptance of Deaf culture in the hearing world, find themselves wishing they were hearing—as a quick solution to an endlessly exasperating problem. Given this double inheritance, who *wouldn't* wish to be free from it?

Chapter 60

What bothers a deaf person the most about hearing people?

▲ What bothers me most is when hearing people think they are complimenting you when they remark, "You are smart for a deaf person," "You did very well for a deaf person," "You speak so well for a deaf person". . . and other variations of the same. Hearing people never compare hearing people this way. This remark automatically shows the false assumption in our society that deaf people are usually inept, not smart, or not on par with hearing people.

D. S.
Northampton, Massachusetts

▲ As a congenitally deaf physician, I have a pet peeve concerning many of my colleagues who constantly use expressions such as "deaf and dumb, weird speech pattern, deaf-mute, talks with gestures," etc., etc.

I take pains to respond to each physician guilty of such entries on medical/surgical charts and/or records and explain that the above-mentioned comments are, at the least, very rude.

I am offering [this example] if you can use it. If nothing else, it makes **me** feel better.

F. H., M.D.
Fremont, California

▲ I can think of many things that are frustrating and irritating, yet I can take them in stride. However, the one thing that upsets me the most is when I am in a group of people, whether friends or family, and a story or joke is told that I cannot understand or has not been interpreted. I ask "What did you just say?", only to be told, "I'll tell you later," with a wave of the hand serving as the only acknowledgement. This not only frustrates me, it makes me feel isolated. This is one of the primary reasons I prefer to be with other deaf people, and those hearing who know ASL & are willing to ensure that all present, deaf or hearing, can be full participants in the group. I have talked with other deaf in my area, and they agree this is also very frustrating. The key here, I think, is to be aware of those around you.

D. E.
Davis, California

▲ What bothers me the most about hearing people is when they are speaking to you and you tell them that you did not understand and mention that you are deaf/ hearing-impaired. They would respond with an "Oh, I am so sorry" and start to speak louder and very slow (very articulate). It makes it harder for me to understand them. It would help if they just spoke normally and did not raise their voice. It would also help if those people were educated about the different kinds of disabilities and how to handle any kind of situations with the handicapped people.

E. M. S.
Newbury Park, California

▲ Easy . . . meeting a hearing person and having their first question be, "Do you speechread?" (of course, expecting me to get that through speechreading). I usually answer, "A little," sometimes answer, "No," and once answered, "I try not to!" (An absurd answer to an absurd question.) It angers me that the attitude is that communication is *my* problem. Without delving too deep—the reason I resist admitting this "speechguessing" ability is that on the occasions before I learned better, I would answer, "Yes" and from then on, they expected 100%, a feat I am not capable of under the best circumstances.

Maybe my next answer should be, "Do you sign?" (in sign only!!)

E. K.
Houston, Texas

Afterword

Above all, please remember that deaf people are human beings. If you treat us like human beings, we will surely reciprocate. There's no telling what the rewards may be.

Also remember: deaf people have dreams, desires, and feelings, just as you do.

Deaf education (and community) in France began with a priest who had compassion for two deaf sisters. Similarly, the American Deaf community began with a father's concern for his deaf daughter and other such children, and a neighbor's interest. A Deaf teacher in Paris agreed to come to the States to teach other deaf people. These individuals helped set into motion a revolution that continues today. They made history. They changed our destiny.

We cannot foresee the possible results of our acts of generosity or simple kindness. Treat a young deaf person with respect, and who knows? Your gesture of encouragement could ultimately result in that person's choosing a career that may have tremendous (and positive) consequences for society. A deaf student could grow up to become the scientist who discovers a cure for AIDS or finds a solution to the ozone problem.

Transforming an oppressed minority into a community of first-class citizens is a mutual task. The bottom line is this: to allow deaf people to have their own community, establish their own identity, fulfill their true potential. We invite you to be part of this adventure.

Select Bibliography

General Reference

Carol Turkington and Allen E. Sussman, Ph.D., **The Encyclopedia of Deafness and Hearing Disorders**. New York: Facts on File, 1992.

John Van Cleve, ed., **Gallaudet Encyclopedia of Deaf People and Deafness**. 3 vols. New York: McGraw-Hill, 1987.

Deaf Culture, Community, and History

Harry Best, **Deafness and the Deaf in the U.S.** New York: Macmillan, 1943.

Jack R. Gannon, **Deaf Heritage: a Narrative History of Deaf America**. Silver Spring, Md.: National Association of the Deaf, 1981.

Nora Ellen Groce, **Everyone Here Spoke Sign Language: Hereditary Deafness on Martha's Vineyard**. Cambridge, Mass.: Harvard University Press, 1985.

Paul C. Higgins, **Outsiders in a Hearing World: A Sociology of Deafness**. Beverly Hills: Sage Publications, 1980.

Mabs Holcomb and Sharon Wood, **Deaf Women: A Parade through the Decades**. San Diego: DawnSignPress, 1989.

Harlan Lane: **When the Mind Hears: A History of the Deaf**. New York: Random House, 1984.

—**The Mask of Benevolence: Disabling the Deaf Community**. New York: Knopf, 1992.

Arden Neisser, **The Other Side of Silence: Sign Language and the Deaf Community in America**. New York: Knopf, 1983. Reprinted with a new introduction, Washington, D.C: Gallaudet University Press, 1990.

Carol Padden and Tom Humphries, **Deaf in America: Voices from a Culture**. Cambridge, Mass.: Harvard University Press, 1988.

Robert Panara and John Panara, **Great Deaf Americans**. Silver Spring, Md.: T.J. Publishers, 1983.

Oliver Sacks, **Seeing Voices: A Journey Into the World of the Deaf**. Berkeley: University of California Press, 1989.

Jerome D. Schein, **At Home Among Strangers**. Washington, D.C.: Gallaudet University Press, 1989.

John Van Cleve and Barry Crouch, **A Place of Their Own: Creating the Deaf Community in America**. Washington, D.C.: Gallaudet University Press, 1989.

Sherman Wilcox, **American Deaf Culture: An Anthology**. Silver Spring, Md.: Linstok Press, 1989.

Richard Winefield, **Never the Twain Shall Meet: The Communications Debate**. Washington, D.C.: Gallaudet University Press, 1987.

Learning Sign Language: Texts and Dictionaries

Dennis Cokely and Charlotte Baker, **American Sign Language: A Student Text** (3 vols.); **A Teacher's Resource Text** (2 vols.). Silver Spring, Md.: T.J. Publishers, 1980.

Elaine Costello, **Signing: How to Speak with Your Hands**. New York: Bantam, 1983.

Tom Humphries, Carol Padden, and Terrence J. O'Rourke, **A Basic Course in American Sign Language**. Silver Spring, Md.: T.J. Publishers, 1980.

Cheri Smith, Ella Mae Lentz, and Ken Mikos, **Signing Naturally**. Vista American Sign Language Series. San Diego: DawnSignPress, 1988.

Families and Other Adventures

Harvey Barash and Eva Barash Dicker, **Our Father Abe: The Story of a Deaf Shoe Repairman**. Madison, Wisc.: Abar Press, 1991.

Bernard Bragg, **Lessons in Laughter: The Autobiography of a Deaf Actor. As Signed to Eugene Bergman**. Washington, D.C.: Gallaudet University Press, 1989.

Lorraine Fletcher, **Ben's Story: A Deaf Child's Right to Sign**. Washington, D.C.: Gallaudet University Press, 1987.

Leo M. Jacobs, **A Deaf Adult Speaks Out**. Washington, D.C.: Gallaudet University Press, 1986.

Frances M. Parsons, **I Didn't Hear the Dragon Roar**. Washington, D.C.: Gallaudet University Press, 1988.

David Wright, **Deafness**. New York: Stein & Day, 1969.

Index
Numbers refer to chapters

If you still have questions...

...send them to us. We welcome your questions and comments. Our feature, "For Hearing People Only," appears every month in **DEAF LIFE**.

Send to:
"For Hearing People Only"
DEAF LIFE
MSM Productions, Ltd.
1095 Meigs St.
Rochester, NY 14620-2405
http://www.deaflife.com

For Hearing People Like what you've been reading? Want to order a copy for yourself, or an extra for a friend?

ONLY

Please print clearly!

Name: _____

Address: _____

City: _____

State: _____ Zip: _____ Phone:(_____) _____

Quantity	Price USA/Outside	Shipping/handling* Regular*	RUSH**	New York Sales Tax	Total
Single copy	$19.95/22.95	☐ $2.00	☐ $5.00	☐ $1.60	
2 copies	$39.95/45.90	☐ $4.00	☐ $5.00	☐ $3.20	
3 copies	$59.85/68.85	☐ $6.00	☐ $5.00	☐ $4.80	
4 copies	$79.80/91.80	☐ $8.00	☐ $5.00	☐ $6.40	

Special quantity discounts (10 or more copies) are available. Contact us for details.

*Regular orders take 2 to 6 weeks for delivery.
**RUSH orders will be sent out within 2 to 4 business days after we receive the order. If you want the book(s) sent via overnight (Express) mail, contact us for details.

Also available in Hardcover format. $35.00 postpaid

**Credit cards (MC, VISA, DC) are accepted ONLY for RUSH orders.

☐ **MasterCard**   ☐ **VISA***   ☐ **DINERS CLUB INTERNATIONAL***

Credit Card #
_/_/_/_/_/_/_/_/_/_/_/_/_/_/_/_/
Expiration date_/_
Signature_____

Canadian/Foreign orders:
Please enclose an International Money Order (**U.S. funds only**).

A $20.00 fine is charged on all bounced checks.

Send this order form with check or money order payable to:
HPO Book, c/o MSM Productions, Ltd.
1095 Meigs Street, Rochester, NY 14620
FAX (716) 442-6371
http://www.deaflife.com
Photocopies of this form accepted.